SHIATSU

ABOUT THE AUTHORS

From the age of 14 Chris Jarmey has studied and practised Hatha Yoga and a variety of martial arts. He has been studying, practising and subsequently teaching Shiatsu since 1970, drawing mainly upon the inspirations of Shizuto Masunaga and Pauline Sasaki. After qualifying in physiotherapy in 1978 he initiated the use of both Shiatsu and therapeutic yoga methods into the hospital environment. Having created a teaching network throughout England and Wales for 'grassroots' Shiatsu, he founded the European Shiatsu School in 1985 as a vehicle for teaching Shiatsu up to practitioner level, with branches throughout Britain and Europe. Chris is the Principal of the European Shiatsu School, and has sat for several terms on the Core Group and Examining Board of the Shiatsu Society.

Gabriel Mojay is a qualified and experienced Shiatsu practitioner, and a registered teacher within the Shiatsu Society. He has also been trained in acupuncture, and is a member of the British Acupuncture Council and register. A qualified medical herbalist, he is Director of the Institute of Traditional Herbal Medicine and Aromatherapy. He has a private practice in Shiatsu, acupuncture, medical herbalism and aromatherapy. Since 1983 Gabriel has taught a variety of approaches to natural healing, including oriental medicine and Shiatsu in particular.

SHIATSU
The complete guide

Chris Jarmey and Gabriel Mojay

Illustrated by Peter Cox
Photography by Peter Warren

Thorsons
An Imprint of HarperCollins*Publishers*

Thorsons
An Imprint of HarperCollins*Publishers*
77–85 Fulham Palace Road
Hammersmith, London W6 8JB

The Thorsons website address is:
www.Thorsons.com

First published by Thorsons 1991
This revised edition 1999

7 9 10 8

© Chris Jarmey and Gabriel Mojay 1991, 1999

Chris Jarmey and Gabriel Mojay assert the moral
right to be identified as the authors of this work

A catalogue record for this book is
available from the British Library

ISBN 0 7225 3914 2

Printed in Great Britain by The Bath Press

Contents

A NOTE ON THE USE OF CAPITALIZATION

Throughout this book you will notice that all words referring to concepts peculiar to Oriental Medicine begin with a capital letter. When the same words describe a more familiar western meaning, they do not. This is standard practice to avoid misrepresentation of meaning. For example, 'Liver' refers to the Oriental medical concept of Liver, whereas 'liver' refers to the anatomical liver organ as understood in western medicine. Other words used in this book such as: Heat, Full, Channel and so on, all have slightly different connotations in Oriental Medicine.

Introduction

WHAT IS SHIATSU?

Shiatsu is a form of bodywork which, at its highest level, combines a finely-tuned intuition with a thorough understanding of the bodymind. Shiatsu was developed in Japan from a synthesis of Chinese massage called Anma and Western techniques of physical manipulation. As a complete system of healing through touch, it draws extensively on key aspects of Traditional Oriental Medicine.

Shiatsu technique involves stretching, holding and leaning body weight into various part of the recipient's body to improve energy flow, blood circulation, flexibility and posture. Pressure and contact is applied through the hands, thumbs, fingers, forearms, knees and feet, with the recipient sitting or lying in various positions. Treatment is focused along specific Channels ('meridians') of subtle bodily energy called Ki. Ki is the life force which sustains every activity of the body, mind and Spirit.

Although Shiatsu literally means 'finger pressure', the spirit of Shiatsu is one of communication through touch. Shiatsu which is responsive to the recipient's needs cannot be achieved by technical skill and intellectual study alone. To be effective, it requires sensitivity in order to feel and positively influence the quality of vitality within the recipient. Vitality is the basis of health, and reflects the strength and harmony of Ki circulation. Shiatsu which is sensitive and supportive both tonifies and corrects the flow of Ki, thereby helping to restore vitality and prevent disease.

To achieve truly supportive Shiatsu, it must be delivered with relaxed body weight and an effortless transmission of Ki. Overt effort from the practitioner will only obstruct Ki flow and prevent the recipient from relaxing and 'opening'. Ki is naturally communicated to the recipient when the practitioner's energy is focused and 'grounded' in the lower belly (the belly is referred to as 'the hara' by Shiatsu practitioners).

Finally, truly accurate Shiatsu therapy depends upon the practitioner's understanding of Traditional Oriental Medicine and its diagnostic skills. A practitioner who is knowledgable will have sufficient confidence to deal with clients suffering from both acute and chronic disorders.

THE HISTORY OF SHIATSU

Although the word Shiatsu was not coined until the early twentieth century, the origins of Shiatsu lie firmly within the roots of Traditional Oriental Medicine. Specifically, it can be traced to China around 530 BC, when Bodhidharma introduced a system of exercises for health and sensory control known as Tao-Yinn. These incorporated a system of self-massage and self-applied pressure point therapy for promoting detoxification and rejuvenation. Tao-Yinn soon became an integral part of the health practices and was gradually exported, along with the other Chinese healing arts, through south-east Asia and Korea.

By the tenth century AD, Chinese Medicine had been introduced into Japan, from which time an amalgam of Vibrational Palm Healing, Spot Pressing and Massage, known collectively as Anma, would have been combined with Tao-Yinn (Do-In) to loosely resemble present day Shiatsu.

Around three hundred years ago, during the Edo era in Japan, doctors were required to study Anma as a means of familiarizing themselves with the human structure, energy channels and pressure points, so that they could accurately diagnose and treat with whatever means they thought appropriate; namely acupuncture, herbs or bodywork. Gradually, however, Anma was reduced to treating simple muscular tensions until by the twentieth century it became licensed only to promote pleasure and comfort.

However, there still existed many Anma therapists who based their work on the original theory, and who coined the name Shiatsu in order to avoid the restrictive regulations applied to Anma. Shiatsu was eventually recognized as a legitimate form of therapy by the Japanese government in the mid-1950s.

Nowadays the official definition given by the Japanese Ministry of Health and Welfare states:

> Shiatsu therapy is a form of manipulation administered by the thumbs, fingers and palms, without the use of any instrument, mechanical or otherwise, to apply pressure to the human skin, to correct internal malfunctioning, promote and maintain health and treat specific diseases.

The Development of Shiatsu in Japan   The official recognition of Shiatsu in Japan can be mainly attributed to the efforts of Tokujiro Namikoshi, who established the Shiatsu Institute of Therapy in Hokkaido in 1925 and the Japan Shiatsu Institute in 1940 (subsequently renamed the Japan Shiatsu School). His success was no doubt due to a combination of his obvious tactile sensitivity and the effort he put into aligning Shiatsu with Western medicine. In this way, his method benefited from the general trend towards Westernization.

The traditional, philosophical and medical framework was reintegrated into Shiatsu by Shizuto Masunaga, who taught at the Japan Shiatsu Institute for ten years before opening his own school known as the Iokai Shiatsu Centre in Tokyo. Also highly developed in tactile sensitivity, Shizuto Masunaga had an interest in integrating the ancient medical model with Western physiology. His main contribution to Shiatsu before his death was to establish the full influence of the major Energy Channels over the surface of the body, and how to fully effect a person's psychological/physical balance through optimum connection with these Channels.

Consequently, in Japan today, there are two distinct methods of Shiatsu: the method developed by Tokujiro Namikoshi, and Iokai Shiatsu as developed by the late Shizuto Masunaga. Namikoshi's style is characterized by applying pressure to specific reflex points which relate to the central and autonomic nervous system, whereas Masunaga's style is characterized by sensitivity to the Energy Channels which are the manifestation of body/mind function, from the viewpoint of Oriental Medicine. Masunaga also introduced the dimension of 'support and connection' by realizing that Shiatsu treatment is much less painful, more nurturing and energetically more effective if both hands are kept apart, yet in contact with the recipient, so that one hand is used as a 'listening' hand, while the other applies technique.

Between the two polarities, there are several Japanese acupuncture schools which teach Shiatsu as a prerequisite to studying acupuncture. Ultimately, however, the effectiveness of Shiatsu depends more upon the attitude, proficiency and attunement of the practitioner, than upon a particular style.

The Development of Shiatsu in the West

Shiatsu did not become widely known in the United States and Europe until the 1970s, although it has been practised by a few Japanese and Occidentals in the West since its conception. Within Europe, Shiatsu has been primarily influenced by the Namikoshi method and the Masunaga method, but with an additional input from macrobiotics[1] which makes use of the traditional Acupuncture Channels and pressure points, plus its own theoretical and philosophical rationale. This method incorporates substantial use of the feet to apply pressure and stretch, commonly known as 'Barefoot' techniques. Shiatsu as practised in Europe is therefore mostly associated with either Masunaga's method (often called Zen Shiatsu), Macrobiotic Shiatsu, Namikoshi method, or various hybrids.

In the United States, Shiatsu had – by the mid 1980s – been classified into the following systems or 'styles':

- *Acupressure Shiatsu*, which focuses specifically upon acupuncture points and encompasses a variety of acupressure styles.
- *Five Element Style Shiatsu*, which relies mainly upon the Five

Element Theory[2] of Traditional Chinese Medicine, especially in relation to the emotions, and which incorporates some macrobiotic principles.

● *Macrobiotic Shiatsu*, which incorporates Classical Acupuncture Channels, Barefoot techniques and the way of living in harmony as advocated by George Ohsawa, Michio Kushi and others.

● *Nippon Style Shiatsu*, which is fundamentally Namikoshi style, and as such places great emphasis on Western physiology, but with the addition of Chinese medical theory and the Classical Energy Channels.

● *Zen Shiatsu*, as developed by Shizuto Masunaga, which is characterized by the application of the Kyo-Jitsu Tonification and Sedation Principle,[3] an extended Energy Channel system, and a condensed synthesis of Traditional Chinese Medicine, Western physiology and psychology.

● *Ohashiatsu*, can also be added to this list as an amalgam of Namikoshi's style with methods developed by Wataru Ohashi, aspects of Zen Shiatsu, and the use of Classical acupoints (Tsubos) and Channels.

It is interesting to observe that in Japan, which has traditionally enjoyed a rich heritage of Traditional Chinese Medicine, the most popular method of Shiatsu first licensed by the Japanese government was the Namikoshi system, which is based upon Western medical concepts to the exclusion of all Traditional Chinese Medical theory and Energy Channels.

Conversely, in both Europe and the United States, all styles of Shiatsu, including those derived from the Namikoshi method, incorporate some aspect of Traditional Oriental Medicine.

1. Macrobiotics is a philosophy of living and eating for harmony and self-development, systemized by George Ohsawa.
2. The Five Elements are fully described in Chapter 10 of this book.
3. Kyo-Jitsu is described extensively throughout this book, see particularly pp.17–19.

PART 1

THE BASICS OF SHIATSU

Shiatsu is a method of bodywork which allows us to give and receive care, warmth and healing through non-intrusive touch. Its potential role within society is forever increasing as we become more divorced from direct personal communication and tactile human contact. Within our industrialized, technological age, there exists a move towards greater human connection and co-operation; Shiatsu will greatly facilitate this.

In this section we will present the basics of Shiatsu necessary to fulfil this need at an appropriate level for use amongst family and friends. These basic principles are, however, equally applicable to Shiatsu as a therapy, and as such should be considered the foundation to Shiatsu practice at all levels.

To appreciate fully the power of Shiatsu, it is necessary at the outset to understand the Oriental concept of energy and its inter-relationship with the human being. To this end, we will firstly define Ki, Channels and Tsubos, and then highlight the difference in emphasis between acupressure and Shiatsu, with a description of Kyo/Jitsu.

Chapter 1

The Concept of Ki

WHAT IS KI?

The difference between that which is living and that which is not living is the relative quantity of what oriental medical tradition speaks of as *Ki* and *Jing*. Ki (Chinese Qi or Ch'i) can be thought of as the power which unifies and animates. It binds energy into matter, which means that without it nothing would hold together and nothing tangible would exist. Ki is therefore a binding, cohesive force at the point where energy is on the verge of materializing, and where matter is at the point of becoming energy. Since matter is itself a form of energy vibration, everything in existence is considered to be Ki. However, it makes for clearer understanding if we limit our interpretation of Ki to be that which animates matter. Therefore beyond its fundamental binding qualities, Ki is also the energy associated with any movement, be it the movement of the sea, wind, blood or of walking. All inanimate and animate things must therefore have Ki to exist, and more Ki to move.

In order to 'live', however, an organism must pass through a process of organic change ranging from birth and growth towards eventual decay. The life essence which makes this possible is known as *Jing* or *Essence*. Jing therefore, is the source of living substance and growth whereas Ki is the ability to bind, activate and move.

However, an organism can exist with sufficient Jing to fulfil its involuntary organic processes and have enough Ki to function, without necessarily exhibiting an indication of consciousness. Consciousness signifies the presence of *Shen*, which is the energy behind the power to think and discriminate, to rationalize and to self reflect. Without Shen, there can be no personality. Ki, Jing and Shen are known in traditional oriental thinking as 'the three Treasures'.

Ki is more widespread than Jing or Shen, because everything we perceive (and much that we do not) has some degree of Ki. Only that which is 'living' in the sense that it is subject to growth, reproduction and decay, has Jing. Only that which is conscious and can self reflect (e.g. humans) has Shen. It is important to realize that Jing and Shen are limited aspects or special manifestations of Ki, as is everything else that exists. Reference to Ki henceforth will refer to its functional aspects of cohesion and movement.

All matter, or in fact anything we can conceptualize, be it a thought or an emotion, has Ki. The difference between the living and the non-living is the presence of Jing, to which Shen may add consciousness. However, Jing and Shen cannot manifest without the cohesive and moving attributes of Ki. The more alive you are, the more Ki you have. An abundance of Ki in a living organism results in high vitality. If a person lacks vitality they will lack the optimum quota of Ki to infuse the Jing and Shen. If they are dead, they are very deficient in Ki (and devoid of Jing and Shen). Decomposition reflects a further depletion until the only Ki remaining is the *minimum* needed to keep the atoms and molecules manifesting as matter. Ki will not produce life, but life is impossible without sufficient Ki.

Ki is everywhere, on and around this earth, although some places have more than others. Moving water generates Ki in abundance, whilst Ki itself is the ultimate source of that movement. This presence of Ki can clearly be appreciated in the proximity of waterfalls and by the sea-shore.

Sunlight is undoubtedly the greatest source of Ki from our perspective. The level of Ki necessary to charge matter with life cannot occur in the absence of sunlight or water. This is obvious with plants, but equally true of animals who can only exist by eating plants or other animals, who themselves feed on plants. Even fungi, which seem to flourish without direct access to sunlight, grow out of material produced by the plants and animals which do.

Sources of Ki in the Body

In order for 'life' to be maintained within our bodies, we must have a constant input of Ki to keep things together and moving. This input is from 3 main sources; initially we inherit it from parents and subsequently we obtain it from air and food. Ki will be explained in greater detail in its relationship to specific oriental medical theory in Part 2 of this book.

WHAT IS A CHANNEL?

Channels – or meridians – are said to be the routes through which Ki flows, forming a network connecting up the Ki associated with all the major functions of the body. The concept of interconnecting Channels is termed *Jing Luo* in Traditional Oriental Medicine. *Jing*[1] means 'to go', 'steer through' or 'to direct', and *Luo* means 'a net', 'network' or 'an attaching system'. We consider *Jing Luo* to carry Ki to all the tissues and organs, whereas Blood is carried within the blood vessels (known as *Xue Mai*). Traditionally, however, the carriage of Ki and Blood within Channels and blood vessels was not precisely differentiated because the

Channels were considered to carry Ki *and* Blood, and blood vessels were considered to carry Blood *and* Ki. To avoid confusion, it is easier to consider the Channels as carrying *only* Ki, although it must be remembered that Ki is the force behind all movement, including the movement of Blood which means that Ki exists in abundance in the blood vessels. Channels can be thought of as 'carrying' Blood in the sense that where the Ki within the Channels is felt to be deficient in a particular body area, there is often an accompanying lack of blood circulation.

Blood vessels and nerves are easy to define because they can be 'seen' to exist, from their precise location upon dissection of the body. We cannot in the same way locate the Channels, which implies they have no physical structure, and do not exist within a dead body.[2] Unlike the electrical wiring of a house which exists whether or not electricity is flowing through it, Channels do not exist independently of Ki. A good comparison is that a beam cannot exist without light. It must be that a Channel and its Ki are one and the same, and exist or cease to exist according to the presence or absence of life.

To help conceptualize a Channel, an analogy can be drawn with water currents. A body of water such as the sea may have specific currents of water flowing through it as a consequence of feeder streams, tidal movements and thermals. However, if the source of these currents is removed by blocking the feeder streams and equalizing the water temperatures throughout, then the course of the deceased water current becomes undetectable. Likewise, the cessation of living functions remove the source of a Channel's existence. A dead body, therefore, has no Ki Channels,[2] in the same way that it has no soul or personality.

You can of course, map out where the surface course of the Channels 'should be' or 'once were' by drawing lines all over the body to match diagrammatic charts. However, this can encourage a 'static' concept of Channel location. In actuality, a Channel's Ki strength and quality will be affected by bodily disharmonies, and its precise location will slightly alter according to variations in Ki flow within adjacent Channels. Again, we can compare this with a water current whose precise location may be altered by variable activity within nearby currents.

Since a Channel may not be quite where it 'should be' according to the map, and since variable factors will alter the exact angle of touch necessary to connect with the Ki, it is essential for the Shiatsu practitioner to develop sensitivity to the continuity of Ki flow in order to maximize the effect of the Shiatsu session.

WHAT IS A TSUBO?

A *Tsubo* is any point along the surface pathway of a Ki Channel where the Ki can be influenced directly by pressure, or by needle insertion. Tsubos are gateways into a person's energetic body and as such, they

Fig. 1.1: Tsubo
The character represents a jar with a narrow neck covered with a lid. The neck represents the Tsubo connecting to the Ki within the Channel represented by the bulbous section of the jar.

can be used to affect the internal environment of a human being.

Acupuncture makes use of those points which have fixed locations. Since they are fixed, these points, when manipulated, have actions on the body and mind which have been recorded empirically for many centuries. A Tsubo does not have to be a fixed and labelled point however, and Shiatsu makes use of those Tsubos which manifest along the Channels *between* the fixed points, as well as the fixed points themselves.

Fixed Tsubos are both energetic vortices where the *normal* or *constant* life processes are relayed to the surface, and where there is an intake or release of Ki between the Channels and the outside world. In contrast, the non-fixed Tsubos are surface reflections of *fluctuating* functional imbalances. The experienced Shiatsu practitioner is able to detect these Tsubos as palpable distortions in the Ki flow of the Channels. In so doing, energy can be tonified if weak, dispersed if in excess or blocked, and calmed if over active, according to the method of touch applied.

Tsubos cannot exist without Ki any more than their Channels can. Both are reactions to the internal environment which is constantly influencing Ki strength and circulation. The energetic outline of a Tsubo is like a vase-shaped vortice with its mouth and neck narrower than its base. The Japanese character for Tsubo illustrates this shape quite accurately.

The experienced Shiatsu practitioner is able to feel the depth and breadth of a Tsubo and feel its response to touch. Also, since everything in the body is connected in some way to everything else, he or she is able to feel resultant reactions in other Tsubos elsewhere in the body.

THE DIFFERENCE BETWEEN SHIATSU AND ACUPRESSURE

Shiatsu can be applied evenly or with variable pressure along the length of Ki Channels. Pressure applied evenly and rhythmically has a smoothing effect on the Ki flow, whereas variable yet stationary pressure, applied according to the level of Ki within the non-fixed Tsubos, will have a deeper effect, because it requires greater focus from the giver.

Most Shiatsu systems are based upon tactile connection with the Ki flowing within the Channels. An exception is the Namikoshi system in Japan which uses neuromuscular physiology as its theoretical basis. Methods which concentrate on the classical 'fixed' Tsubos for their specific reactions upon the body and mind are known as Acupressure. In contrast, Shiatsu focuses less upon the classical Tsubos and more upon the Channel pathways themselves.

Acupressure is generally geared to relieving the recipient's suffering by tonifying weak Ki, calming overactive Ki, or dispersing blocked Ki via the classical Tsubos. Systems which emphasize the classical Tsubos often view deficient Ki as an independent phenomenon from excess Ki, and vice versa. Shiatsu differs in so far as it deals more with the interaction between Ki Channels, viewing excess or deficiency as distortions in the energetic web of Ki flow. Therefore it is recognized that excess Ki within one Tsubo often requires a relative deficiency within another. If a Channel has predominantly excess Ki, then another must be relatively deficient. Channel imbalances are therefore seen as reflecting relative distortions within the person as a whole. Shiatsu is based upon rectifying Channel distortions. However, most Shiatsu systems incorporate some acupressure technique.

KYO JITSU

Assessing and balancing interacting Channel distortions is highly developed in the Zen Shiatsu system. Shizuto Masunaga referred to depleted, empty or underactive Ki as *Kyo*, and excess, full or hyperactive Ki as *Jitsu*. Both Kyo and Jitsu refer to relative states of emptiness and fullness, and therefore do not exist or mean anything in the absence of the other. Masunaga draws the analogy of Kyo/Jitsu distortion with vector distortions in a ball. From Fig. 1.2 we can see that the empty, depressed Kyo area gives rise to the full, protruding Jitsu area.

You can expect any Channel to err towards Kyo or Jitsu in relation to any other. The whole pattern is constantly fluctuating. The aim of Shiatsu is to discover the root cause behind any acute or chronic disharmony and attempt to stabilize it. The Jitsu areas are easy to find because they exhibit activity and protrude from the surface. They are however, only the result of deeper weakness, less obviously exhibited as Kyo elsewhere.

The most direct and surest way to balance overall Kyo/Jitsu distortions and therefore allow the body/mind its optimum potential for healing is to find the most Kyo Channel and balance it off against the Channel which is most Jitsu. All the other minor imbalances in the other Channels will tend to equalize as a result.

The emptying or moving of Jitsu is referred to as *sedation* or *dispersal*, whereas the filling and strengthening of Kyo is referred to as *tonification*. It is essential that Kyo/Jitsu is accurately assessed, and that a recipient who is generally weak is not further weakened by the overuse of dispersal techniques. This can easily occur because Jitsu is much easier to locate within the body than Kyo. Each Channel exhibits differing degrees of Kyo/Jitsu emphasis throughout its own pathway, so that once the most Kyo and most Jitsu Channels have been located, each must be dealt with according to their energetic presentation. The most profound part of a treatment will be the tonification of the weakest Tsubos within the weakest area of the weakest Channel.

The principle methods of tonifying Kyo and dispersing Jitsu are fully explained in Chapter 3 (p.34).

Fig. 1.2: Kyo/Jitsu

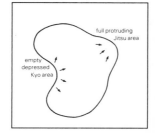

Comparison of Kyo/Jitsu

Kyo	*Jitsu*
Below surface	Protruding from surface
Less obvious	More obvious
Passive resistance or no resistance	Active resistance
Empty – requires filling	Full – requires emptying/dispersing
Underactive, leading to stiffness or flaccidity	Hyperactive, leading to congestion, blockage and impenetrability
Slower to respond	Immediate response
Underlying cause	Manifests as symptoms
Requires deep, sustained connection	Requires light, superficial connection, or none at all
Its tonification affects the whole person	Its dispersal affects localized body areas

Both Kyo and Jitsu can feel hard and unyielding to touch, which can confuse the inexperienced practitioner. Kyo can have the impenetrable feeling of a solid, locked door to an empty room. The impenetrability of Jitsu, however, is analogous to the sheer volume of people within a room who can do without your presence to add to the squeeze. Ki however, is more tenuous than crowds of people, so it takes a degree of subtlety and awareness to detect its measure.

A useful analogy can be drawn from knocking on the doors of houses in a street:

a. Some reveal an obvious presence because someone answers the door (Ki is clearly present);
b. The person who answers the door may aggressively send you away (Extreme Jitsu);
c. They may open the door before you knock and send you away (Very extreme Jitsu);
d. Someone opens the door out of curiosity and allows you into the lobby, if you are pleasant to them (Neutral);
e. Someone answers the door, is lonely and desperate for company, so encourages you to come in (Acute Kyo);
f. Nobody is in and the door is wide open (Flaccid Kyo);
g. Nobody is in, but the door is double-bolted for security (Chronic stiff Kyo).

From this analogy we can see that the attitude and approach of the caller is important. A very aggressive caller (or Shiatsu technique) might succeed in forcing their way in where they are not welcome, causing pain and a great deal of discord in the neighbourhood (which is analogous to the body/mind). The same caller might overstep the hospitality of those desperate for company, causing tension as a defensive reaction. A particularly insensitive and aggressive 'caller' might smash down the bolted door to get 'results' and thus cause permanent damage.

Aggression and insensitivity are therefore the antithesis of gaining safe and welcome entry into both house and Tsubo. Sensitivity and patience is required in all circumstances.

Recognizing degrees of deficiency within the chronic stiff Kyo areas requires almost ethereal subtlety. It can be done quite easily with practice if you again think of Ki within a Tsubo as similar to people within a house. When you knock on enough doors you develop a sense of *knowing* when nobody is in, or when somebody is *pretending* not to be in, even though both seem to be empty at first glance. In Kyo Tsubos you are therefore tuning your senses to the detection of a presence, even if it does not want to show itself. When you have found it, you can offer it your support.

1. *Jing* – not to be confused with the term 'Jing' meaning 'Essence' in another context.
2. Channels, however, do seem to affect the tissues through which they pass, with changes that persist even after death. Research in China led by Professor Zhu Zong Xiang from Beijing shows that the skin is thinner along the Channels than it is adjacent to them. He also discovered that infrasonic waves travel more quickly and with a higher pitch along Channel pathways than in surrounding areas. Professor Zhang Baozhen has also found that nerve endings are more expanded along the course of major Channels compared to elsewhere.

Chapter 2

The Essentials of Competent Shiatsu

The basic aims of Shiatsu for use at a grassroots level amongst family and friends are:

- To help the recipient relax and therefore provide a means to combat the effects of stress;
- To improve the recipient's lymphatic flow, blood circulation and vitality (and therefore boost the immune system);
- To help alleviate aches, pains and stiffness;
- To help both the giver and receiver become more aware of their bodies;
- To develop healing compassion through appropriate physical contact.

These aims are most readily achieved if the giver of Shiatsu applies the essential ingredients of Shiatsu, which are:

- Motivation
- Steadiness of breath
- Strong and open Hara
- Relaxation and comfort
- Empty Mind
- Support rather than force
- Positive connection
- Perpendicular pressure
- Stationary pressure
- Technical ability
- Continuity
- Fluency
- Empathy

MOTIVATION

To give Shiatsu there must be a genuine desire to help people feel better. If this desire is absent then there can be no sincere motivation for being involved with this humanitarian healing art.

It is interesting that the written character for 'human' in Japanese embodies the Shiatsu qualities of support and connection, which are fundamental qualities of the human ideal.

You will find that giving Shiatsu makes you feel better, more grounded and more open both physically and energetically, because the more you give of yourself in the service of humankind, the more universal Ki will come flooding back in. This is because nature hates empty spaces. The motivation for giving Shiatsu should be to help others, thereby helping yourself.

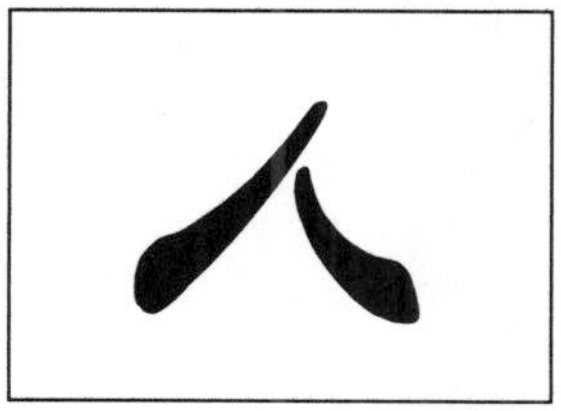

STEADINESS OF BREATH

The breath is intimately connected to thought processes, insofar as deep relaxed breathing produces equanimity of mind and vice versa. Scattered, unfocused thoughts are usually reflected in shallow, irregular breathing, whereas focused attention of the mind only manifests when the breath has slowed to a point where there is a natural period of 'no breathing' between exhalation and inhalation. This can be demonstrated by asking someone to drop a pin somewhere out of sight but within earshot. Listening for the almost imperceptible sound of the pin drop requires such focused attention that the breath stops momentarily. The ability to listen for a pin drop amongst intense distractions fighting for the attention of the mind and emotions is an example of being 'centred'. Centredness is therefore proportional to steadiness of breath, while erratic, shallow breath is symptomatic of those who are not grounded. For the giver of Shiatsu, being 'centred' means being able to feel the barely perceptible changes in muscle tone, circulation and energy levels, as well as having the sensitivity to tune into the recipient's frame of mind; it is knowing when the recipient's tensions relax both physically and mentally. One is truly centred if all this can be achieved irrespective of ongoing personal conflicts and all other distractions.

Fig. 2.1: The Japanese Character for Human; each stem is clearly supporting the other. Mutual support is achieved by leaning and relaxing rather than tensing and pushing

STRONG AND OPEN HARA

Increased centredness can be achieved in many ways. Most spiritual disciplines, if they are practised sincerely, will be of great value, but more especially if there is some emphasis on drawing the mind to the belly, which is the actual physical centre of the body, known as the *Hara*. The energetic centre and physical pivot point of the Hara is known as the *Tanden*, which is located below the navel in the lower abdomen. Aikido, Qi-Qong, Tai-Chi, Yoga, Zen and various meditation methods are all excellent for developing Hara strength and awareness. Focusing energy in the Hara harmonizes the body, mind emotions and spirit, which enables us to harmonize with our surroundings and to react positively to the needs of those receiving Shiatsu.

When we describe someone as 'coming from their Hara', we are describing somebody who is well grounded, strongly focused and using the maximum potential of their body and mind together. In the case of a purely physical movement such as sawing a piece of wood, the person

Fig. 2.2: Hara

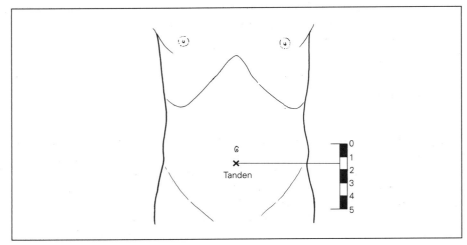

focused in Hara will use strength from their Hara, by focusing the mind and breath there, so that all the movements necessary to saw the wood will derive from the Hara. In contrast, the person who is not centred in Hara will saw the wood by focusing the breath in the chest and utilize excessive tension and strength from the arms and shoulders.

It is essential that all our movements and techniques in Shiatsu originate from the Hara. Indeed, the proper practice of Shiatsu itself encourages Hara development and centring. Underlying *all* Shiatsu technique is Hara. Diagram 'A' illustrates someone applying pressure with no strength of consciousness in Hara, who is thus forced to use upper body strength. Contrast this with Diagram 'B' which illustrates pressure applied by body weight alone.

For maximum use of Hara it is essential to *keep a low centre of gravity*. This will ensure maximum stability for the giver, and allow the

Fig. 2.3(a): Below Pressure applied with upper body strength

Fig. 2.3(b): Below right Pressure applied with body weight alone

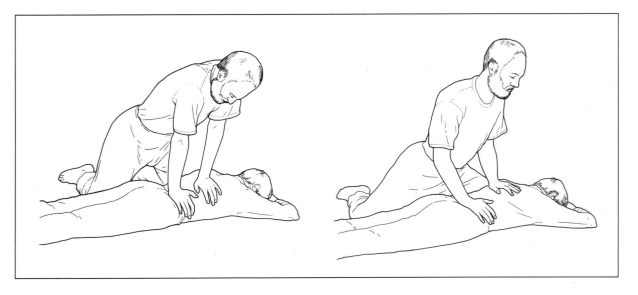

neck, shoulders and muscles of the back to relax. When the centre of gravity is too high, the postural muscles must overwork in order to maintain a steady position, resulting in early fatigue.

A low centre of gravity can be maintained by;

- Keeping the knees and hips spread open.
- Keeping the Hara relaxed – to allow natural, deep breathing.
- Directing the mind and breath to Tanden – rather than allowing the concentration of thought to disperse.
- Keeping weight underside – this can be achieved by imagining all the weight of the body accumulating on the undersurfaces. For example, underside of forearms, underside of belly and so on (see Fig. 2.6).

Once a low centre of gravity has been achieved and can be maintained, it is possible for all movements to originate from, and feel connected to, Tanden.

RELAXATION AND COMFORT

If you are tensed up and unable to relax as a giver of Shiatsu, work on it by developing Hara to steady the mind and breath. When you are in actual physical contact with another being, they will consciously or subconsciously know the degree of tension or relaxation in you, because it will be transmitted to them through your touch. Tension and relaxation are infectious. Have you noticed how relaxing it is to have a cat on your lap? Much more so than having a tense and awkward person work on your shoulders! You can only be truly relaxed if you are

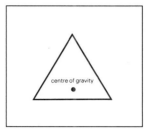

Fig. 2.4: Low centre of gravity (stable)

Fig. 2.5: High centre of gravity (unstable)

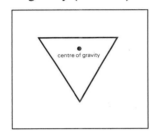

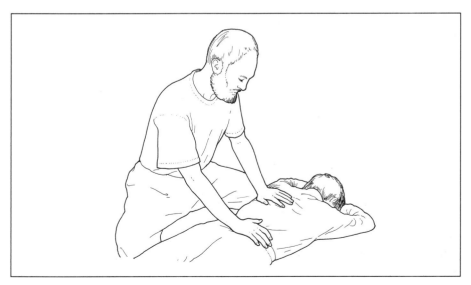

Fig. 2.6: Practitioner imagines weight on undersurfaces of body, i.e. palms, lower forearms, lower belly, lower legs, in order to keep a low centre of gravity.

Fig. 2.7: Comfort and ease of position of giver

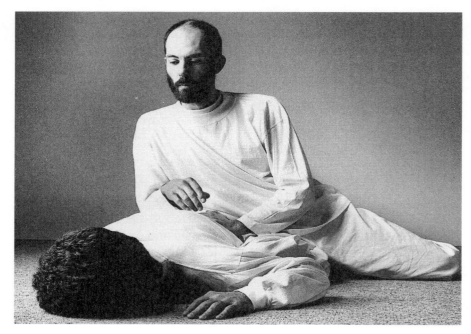

comfortable, so abandon all dramatic and contorted positions even if they do look impressive, and just get comfortable.

Good Shiatsu can relax someone no matter where they are, but if it can be done in quiet, pleasant, amenable surroundings, so much the better. For both giver and receiver, having an empty stomach without being ravenously hungry, wearing loose cotton rather than statically charged, clingy, artificial materials, avoiding fluorescent lighting and concentrations of electrically-operated devices, will all add to comfort as well as promoting maximum energy levels.

EMPTY MIND

Once steadiness in mind and breath has been achieved, and you are firmly established in Hara, then you can apply Shiatsu with what is known as *Empty Mind*.

Shiatsu is much more about feeling than thinking. If you are constantly thinking what you should be feeling, you will probably feel nothing other than a bag of flesh and bones, and be perplexed as to what to do with it. Also, if you are constantly thinking of what you should be doing, your recipient will be constantly wondering what is going to be done to them. Only by keeping our head 'out of the way', so that our awareness is in our Hara, will we be guided by limitless intuition rather than intellect, which is limited. Thinking is a valid and necessary process in a Shiatsu health assessment, but basic Shiatsu is the natural act of touching and holding another human being, and as such pre-empts thinking. Shiatsu touch does not actually require learning as much as relearning and unlearning poor postural habits and responses. If you have difficulty with this, let a baby or a cat crawl over your back and experience natural basic Shiatsu!

SUPPORT RATHER THAN FORCE

The whole purpose of Shiatsu is to encourage a free flow of energy throughout the body and mind. Where there is tension, there is constriction and consequent restriction of blood and energy circulation. Where there is relaxation, there is 'opening' and consequent free flow of blood and vitality. If we push and poke at our fellow human beings, whether physically or verbally, we meet with resistance as they close up, fight back or withdraw. If we support them they will feel secure, have trust and become receptive to our presence.

The first level of support is therefore to project the idea that you are going to *assist* your recipient rather than impose something upon them.

The second level of support is to ensure stability. The most stable

Leg positions for sidelying

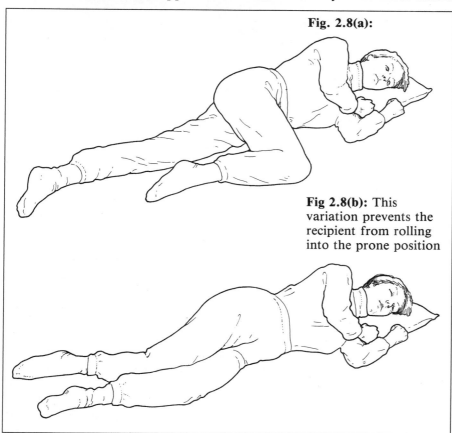

Fig. 2.8(a):

Fig 2.8(b): This variation prevents the recipient from rolling into the prone position

SHIATSU

Fig. 2.9: Bodily
contact for support in
sitting

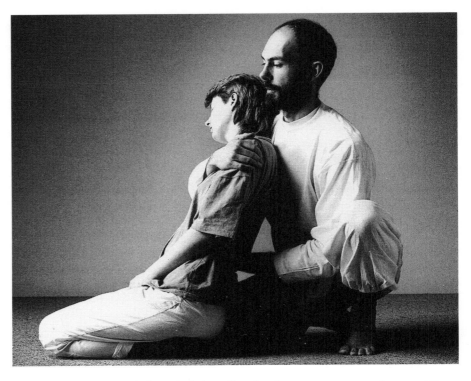

position for the recipient is lying flat in the prone or supine position, whereupon the floor is providing maximum support for the entire body. In this position, no muscular tension is required to offset the effect of gravity upon the posture, unlike in sitting or standing, both of which prohibit total relaxation because the postural muscles remain active.

In sidelying, it is generally beneficial to add support for the head by adding a pillow, and positioning the legs in such a way that prevents a gradual collapsing into prone (see Fig. 2.8).

Basically, the more vertical the recipient's position is for Shiatsu, the more body contact you should give to counteract the force of gravity. Sitting Shiatsu therefore requires maximum body contact to prevent collapse (see Fig. 2.9).

However, total support may not be desirable in every situation. Sometimes you may want to encourage the recipient to 'meet you halfway', especially if you feel they could benefit from gradually taking more responsibility for themselves and be less reliant on others. Part of the art of Shiatsu is to gauge how much support to give. Too much contact and support can be smothering to some people.

The third level of support is the supportive touch. Assuming they are not going to fall over when you apply some of your weight, they may still react defensively if you push or press. By initiating your movement from Hara, and *leaning* rather than pushing, your touch will be welcomed rather than repelled. Consequently the recipient will open up rather than close.

It is the earth which ultimately supports everything in our life, and the closest we can get to the earth is to lie flat on the ground. This is one reason why Shiatsu is better done on the floor rather than on a table. Also, the more grounded we are as givers of Shiatsu, the more support we can give. Once more, good Hara is the key.

Finally, the fourth level of support is to be accessible if the receiver needs to clarify any after-effects arising out of a Shiatsu session, in which case a supportive word from you at the right time will put their mind at ease.

POSITIVE CONNECTION

Connection is really an extension of support. You cannot support somebody unless you are in some way connected to them, yet you can connect with somebody in such a way as to undermine their support; for example, by physically pushing them over, or by making some verbal connection that undermines their confidence, trust and optimism. Consequently, connection can be positive or negative, and as givers of Shiatsu we have the opportunity to enhance positive connection.

Positive connection has both a physical and psychological aspect, which together form the strongest possible energetic connection. The first opportunity to be positively connected is to be open and friendly and to deliberately seek some area of common ground between yourself and the recipient. This should be aimed for as soon as you meet or speak to the recipient, although it will probably be achieved already with those recipients who are family or friends.

On the physical level, the touch of one finger or thumb on a remote part of the body, compared to simultaneous touch from two hands, is very different. When two hands consciously contact the recipient a circuit is completed giving a sense of unification between the giver and receiver, and between the two hands in contact. Touching with only one hand however, is much more likely to result in a feeling of intrusion, or at best localized soothing.

What works best, with a few exceptions, is to have both hands in contact with the person, but kept slightly apart, rather than one on top of the other. The giver should then focus on Hara rather than on hands or thumbs. This will result in the receiver experiencing the two contact places as if they were one large single area of contact. If sustained longer, the receiver will experience the sensation of a single unified contact deep within their being. Meanwhile, the giver will experience this as a distinct current of energy or 'echo' between the two hands. This may feel like a circle of continuity through and with the receiver, between the hands and through one's own Hara. A truly experienced practitioner can maintain this sensation when one hand is stationary and the other is moving, which greatly enhances the quality of continuity, as discussed later.

PERPENDICULAR PRESSURE

Since Shiatsu is concerned with harmonizing Ki, it is important that pressure, whether applied with palms, fingers, thumbs or whatever, is applied at right angles to the surface of the body. This is because the surface distortion caused by non-perpendicular pressure tends to compress and stretch the tissues unevenly around the point of contact. This is very good for increasing blood circulation and lymphatic drainage, but does not have sufficient energetic penetration to make a direct connection with the Ki within the Channels. Instead it may encourage its random dispersal. If a person is very weak and deficient in Ki, this method could upset the delicate interplay of Ki still further, and cause the recipient to become even more deficient. Although rubbing and shaking techniques can be useful as a general warm up for the muscles and a 'loosener' for the joints, one should generally avoid overdoing this with the weak, chronically Ki-deficient person.

Perpendicular pressure produces a 'centring' quality by creating a steady, even epicentre of contact, which has a magnetic attraction to Ki, and is therefore very tonifying for that area if held for several seconds.

Perpendicular penetration is even more crucial when connecting directly with a Tsubo. Since a Tsubo is shaped like a vase, non-perpendicular contact will fail to get beyond its neck, and therefore make little or no contact with Channel Ki, unless the Tsubo is Jitsu, and Ki is blocked in the neck of that Tsubo.

For the receiver, the feeling of incorrectly angled contact will be like superficial manipulation of the surface of the body, which after a short time can become tedious. Off-centre, deep physical pressure can feel very irritating, painful and invasive. Deep connection is determined purely by focus, angle and awareness centred in Hara, and has nothing to do with how hard the Tsubo is physically pressed. In fact, too much physical pressure merely causes defensive reactions which block Ki connection.

Practise accurate perpendicular connection with Tsubos. It is not difficult to master with a little time and patience. Without some sensitivity in this area, the effect of your Shiatsu will be severely impaired.

Fig. 2.10: Dispersal quality of non-perpendicular pressure, compared to 'magnetic' tonifying quality of perpendicular pressure

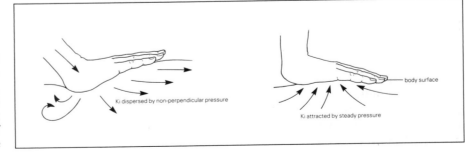

STATIONARY PRESSURE

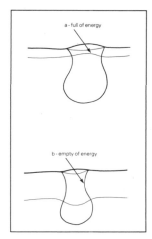

Because the deepest Shiatsu treatment is the tonification of the deficient Kyo Tsubos, it is essential to understand that stationary pressure will be used more frequently than variable pressure techniques. Stationary pressure is deeply penetrating and therefore able to connect with deficient Ki which lies more deeply below the surface than excess Ki. Also, sustained pressure calms the internal organs by stimulating the parasympathetic nervous system. Two to ten seconds of pressure generally suffices, although up to forty-five seconds is sometimes required. In general, stationary perpendicular pressure is the main method of tonifying the Kyo, whereas non-perpendicular techniques such as shaking, circling, rocking, kneading, or anything which involves more movement will sedate or disperse Jitsu. Remember however, that *no* lasting sedation of Jitsu will be achieved unless the Kyo that caused it has been tonified. Various techniques are described in Chapter 3.

Fig. 2.11: Non-perpendicular pressure may connect with a Tsubo full of energy, but fail to make any connection with one that is more empty

TECHNICAL ABILITY

To give Shiatsu you must have a repertoire of techniques to draw upon. If you are a beginner you will find it easier to stick to a regular sequence of techniques. With more experience you will gain the confidence to select appropriate techniques to suit the recipient's unique energetic imbalances and eventually be able to create or adapt techniques to fit any given circumstance. All that is required is constant diligent practice.

Actually, your skill as a practitioner is not a reflection of how many techniques you know, but of your proficiency in delivering them well. It is best to learn a few fundamental techniques for the face up, face down, side lying and sitting positions. Experience will automatically present more advanced variations if all the principles of Shiatsu described in this chapter are integrated into your work. Quality rather than quantity is the key.

Avoid the egocentricity of 'performing' Shiatsu. It is possible to look very gymnastic and dextrous with your technique, but if that is your reason for doing it, the therapeutic value of your session will be severely diminished. This is because the more you are concerned with how you look and rate in the eyes of the recipient, the less you will be able to focus upon them. Consequently, the less you will be able to help them, because sensitivity to Ki gathers where your consciousness is directed. For this reason empathy and Ki sensitivity are inversely proportional to egocentricity.

Fig. 2.12: Pressure on the neck of a deficient Tsubo may create distortions detrimental to Ki flow

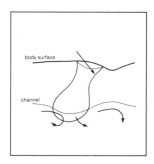

CONTINUITY

To receive good Shiatsu is to experience a feeling of integration throughout the body and between the body and mind. This only happens however, if there is a sense of connection, support and continuity from the giver. A session should therefore be conducted in a co-ordinated flowing manner rather than as a disjointed amalgam of random techniques. Each technique should be a logical extension of the previous one, and wherever possible, contact should be maintained as the hand moves from one area to the next. For example, if the thumb is applied to area A, then B, then C, the hand should glide over the surface between A, B and C, rather than taking it away from the body each time (see Fig. 2.13). Making and breaking contact continuously will inhibit the receiver's ability to relax to deeper levels, because they will be unsure where the contact will be felt next, or perhaps they will try to anticipate your movements upon them. What we want is for them to experience the 'now' because of the reality of contact is only in the present.

Just consider, if you the giver do not know where you are going or why, the receiver is hardly going to be overwhelmed with confidence in you (see Fig. 2.14).

CHANNEL CONTINUITY

Shiatsu not only makes use of the fixed acupuncture points, but also uses those transient Tsubos which manifest elsewhere along a Channel. Consequently, it is possible to work on an entire Channel rather than on the classical acupoints alone. By keeping a support hand stationary, and

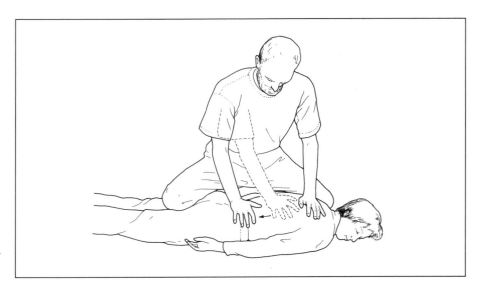

Fig. 2.13: Hand glides over body area between points of pressure

the other hand working along the course of a Channel, we begin to feel points which react to our presence, either directly in the moving hand, indirectly in the support hand, or in both hands. By feeling reactions between both the support and moving hands, we begin to experience the energetic quality of the Channel, therefore enabling us to follow its course via the Tsubos that appear within it, tonifying, dispersing or calming them as required. This is known as 'Channel Continuity' because the pattern of where and when the body is touched is based upon sensitivity and connection to the Channel's flow throughout its whole length, or sections of its length, rather than solely upon the actions of individual classical points.

FLUENCY

Fluency means being well practised in a wide variety of techniques. It is the ability to give a full body Shiatsu, or a specific treatment without having to think about technique. When a language is spoken fluently, one does not have to search so hard for words to express what one wants to say. Likewise, when a Shiatsu practitioner wants to produce a particular effect, the techniques should manifest of themselves.

Fluency is only possible through repeated practice. For the beginner it is best to practise set technique sequences so that the need to decide what to do next is eliminated. This will leave more space for developing touch qualities.

For the giver of Shiatsu, fluency frees the mind to remain in the 'now', which is the only time and place where the receiver's level of vitality can be perceived through touch. The 'now' is missed if the mind

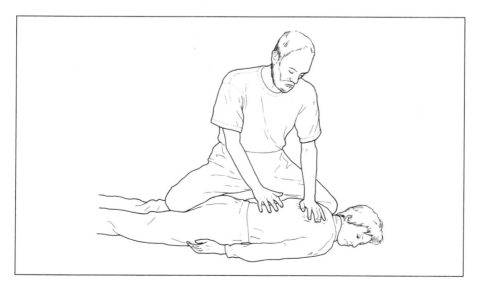

Fig. 2.14: Making and breaking contact leaves the recipient anticipating or bewildered as to where you will touch next

is locked in the past trying to remember relevant techniques to suit the occasion.

Another important aspect of Shiatsu fluency is the ability to move from one part of the body to another with minimal effort and disturbance, especially where it involves moving from one side of the recipient to the other. This is known as *transitioning*.

A good transition is when the giver has moved without the receiver noticing. Many Shiatsu sessions have compromised their relaxing benefits because the giver has fumbled about changing positions without having given due consideration to this aspect of their practice.

EMPATHY

Empathy is the ability and inclination to appreciate how another person is feeling. The strongest form of empathy is in the ability to actually 'feel' how another person is feeling. The two ingredients which enhance empathy are focus in Hara and genuine concern for the other's well-being. Really, these two ingredients need to be united for full effect. Genuine concern is reflected in the level of openness in your heart. This openness, when anchored to a grounded sense of Hara, enables the giver to put him or herself in the position of the receiver and sympathize with them. If heart only is involved, the giver could easily become thrown off-centre by over-sympathizing with any strong emotions exhibited by the recipient. The grounding from Hara however, will give a degree of objectivity and consequent clarity.

What happens if you give Shiatsu with strong Hara but a closed heart is that you may pick up the general level of vitality, but have no sense of their emotional needs. Without the element of compassion, there could also be an inclination towards heavy-handed techniques which could produce unnecessary physical pain.

If the heart is open, but the Hara is closed, the giver will use too much energy through inefficient application of body weight. More significantly, the giver will give too much of his or herself emotionally and energetically without harvesting the limitless universal Ki which can be channelled through one's body by connecting heart to Hara.

Chapter 3

The Tools of Shiatsu

No special equipment is required to give Shiatsu. All you need is your body, plus enough clean floor space for the recipient to lie down, and for you to move around them. The floor should be comfortable but firm. A futon one or two layers thick is ideal, although a thick carpet covered with a sheet will suffice. A thin cotton or silk cloth approximately 18″ square is useful for applying techniques to the neck and face, because Shiatsu feels better and is less obtrusive through a barrier of thin natural fibres. Technique applied to bare skin tends to be more superficial because the sensation of skin contact distracts from feeling the deeper and more subtle presence of Ki. The superficial sensory nerve endings are most prolific on the surface, so a cloth barrier will dampen down the surface tactile sensations and allow the receiver to feel the deeper connection.

For this reason it is essential that the receiver is completely covered in a single layer of clothing throughout the session. This has the added advantage of making sexual innuendo and embarrassment less likely to manifest. Also it means that Shiatsu can be given almost anywhere. Even in the office, Shiatsu to the head, neck and shoulders can be applied.

It might seem from first impressions that a Tsubo would be easier to find and feel on bare skin, but a little practice through thin cloth reveals this to be untrue.

GENERAL PRINCIPLES OF TONIFYING, DISPERSING, AND CALMING KI

Tonifying   To tonify Ki, apply stationary pressure with a thumb or fingertip perpendicular to the mouth of the Tsubo, so that a deep connection can be made. Hold the pressure until you feel some reaction there. Sometimes it feels like the vase shaped Tsubo is filling up with Ki. This should take from about ten seconds to four minutes. If you feel nothing after four minutes, move on to another Tsubo, perhaps returning later to the ones which are slow to react.

It is important that the pressure is not too deep as this could have the counterproductive effect of dispersing Ki, as well as feeling invasive and painful to the recipient. You should go into the Tsubo with the attitude of *meeting* the Ki. Remember that Ki goes where the mind is focused. Therefore, you can be more effective with less pressure if you clearly *visualize* the area lying slightly deep to your finger's depth of penetration. In this way, the recipient's Ki will be drawn to meet your Ki, which will be projected slightly ahead of your fingertip. If and when a connection is felt, reduce the pressure slightly to allow Ki to fill the Tsubo.

This principle of 'Ki attraction' can be compared to touching the surface of water with the tip of your finger. The surface tension of water allows itself to be drawn up by your fingertips, so that as you slowly pull your finger away, the water follows. However, unlike water, a new level of Ki will persist in the Tsubo even after the finger has been removed. That is why the more sensitive and focused the practitioner becomes, the less pressure need be applied. Consequently, a recipient in the hands of an experienced practitioner will experience a deep connection from a relatively light touch.

With practice, sensitivity and a great deal of focus, broad tonification of an area can also be achieved with palms, elbows, knees or feet.

Dispersing

As we have indicated, it is possible to disperse (or sedate) Ki by deeply penetrating a Jitsu Tsubo. However, this is invasive and painful and can be likened to dispersing a crowd with a baton charge; dispersal is achieved but nobody is very happy as a result.

The reason for using a dispersal technique is to unblock a concentration of Ki so that it can move smoothly along the Channel. To achieve this, you can ease your thumb or finger a little way into the Tsubo, and apply a rotatory movement, imagining the Ki being loosened and dispersed. Then, progressively ease the pressure, so that you spiral out of the point. Alternatively, 'pumping' in and out of a mildly Jitsu Tsubo is sometimes effective.

It is worth remembering that a firm support hand on a nearby Kyo area will usually speed up dispersal from the Jitsu region, as well as minimize pain. However, if an area is very full, these dispersal techniques can create too much pain. Extremely full areas are best left alone, because if you develop enough skill in finding and tonifying Kyo areas, the Jitsu areas will often react by dispersing spontaneously.

Stretching, squeezing and shaking techniques all effectively disperse areas which are generally Jitsu.

Calming

Calming is a gentler type of dispersal. Sometimes an area of the body, or a Tsubo, presents a Jitsu quality because the Ki in that area is hyperactive, rather than too concentrated. In this situation, a calming technique is indicated. Calming is achieved by simply covering the area with your palms and remaining calm and peaceful yourself. Do exactly what you would do if you were trying to calm an anxious or upset friend; keep centred and apply a supportive touch.

It sometimes happens that a very hysterical person is calmed with a slap. Slapping a 'hysterical' area of the body (not the head) also works in Shiatsu, but you must be **very** experienced and confident in your abilities to try this technique. A gentle stroking action along a Channel is also very calming. However, remember that nothing you do will be calming if you, the practitioner are not calm and centred yourself.

The parts of the body which can be used to apply technique are:

- Palms
- Thumbs
- Fingers
- Elbows
- Knees
- Feet

PALMS

Although less specific than the fingertips or thumbs, the palms are more soothing, with less potential for causing pain or damage. The whole surface area of the palm should be kept in full contact with the recipient so that the hand can mould around the contours of the body. The palms will therefore lie more flat on the back, or curl to envelop an arm or an ankle. The palms and fingers must remain relaxed (see Fig. 3.1).

Arms should remain outstretched, but with the elbows unlocked. The angle of the body in relation to the arms will determine the amount of pressure applied (see Fig. 3.2).

When closer body contact is preferred, it is sometimes useful to have the arms angled 90° at the elbow, with the knee or inner thigh

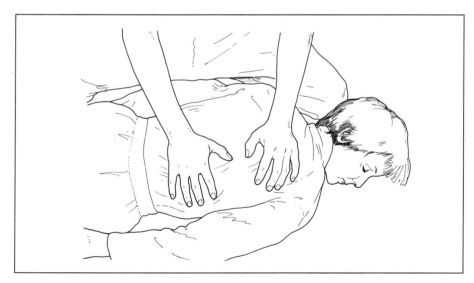

Fig. 3.1: Palms and
fingers relaxed

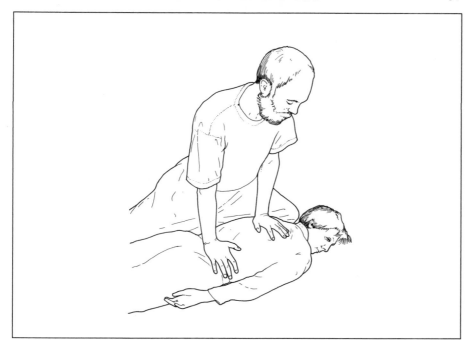

Fig. 3.2: Angle of body in relation to arms

supporting your upper arm. There is however a slight reduction in the connection of Ki flow between Hara and palms with this method (see Fig. 3.3).

Keeping both hands in contact but spread apart is the most therapeutic method because of the increased connection and support. This method enables one hand to 'listen' while the other hand is active, or allows one to tonify while the other calms or disperses.

Support Hand Technique

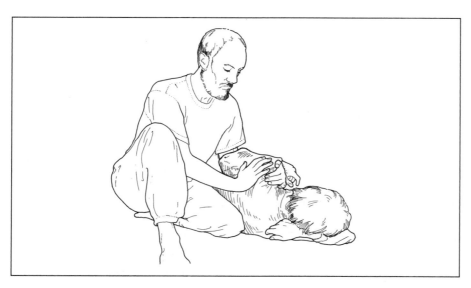

Fig. 3.3: Arms angled 90° at elbow

Fig. 3.4: Support hand technique: tonifying hand should be applied at right angles

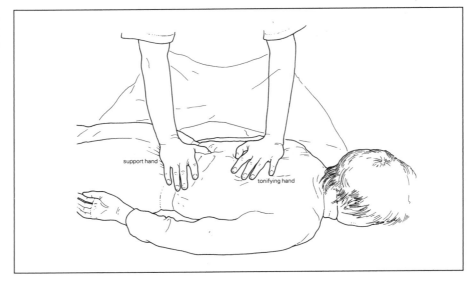

Fig. 3.5: Hands lying one on top of the other

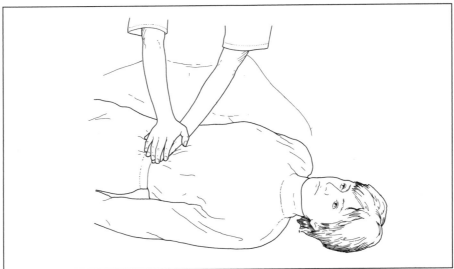

Palm Overlap Technique   Hands lying one on top of the other can be used when a malleable 'wave like' action is required.

Circular Rotations/Shaking   Although more superficial in effect than focused, stationary, perpendicular pressure, rotations and shaking are especially effective for relieving muscular tensions around the shoulder blades, or for stimulating warmth in the pelvic region when applied to the sacrum. Note that the connective tissues should be moved over the underlying bone rather than merely frictioning the surface.

Grasping   This method is especially useful when applied to the arms and legs. One

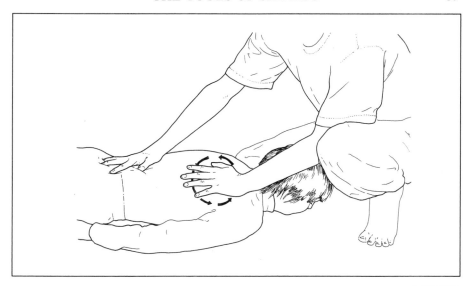

Fig. 3.6: Circular rotations on shoulder blades

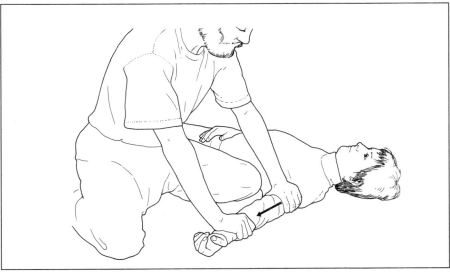

Fig. 3.7: One hand clasps limb for support, other moves along limb

hand clasps the limb for support, while the other moves along the limb. A firm support hand is very important.

With fingers interlocked, pressure is applied simultaneously with the heels of both hands. This method is used to squeeze the muscles either side of the lumbar spine, from the kidney region down to the pelvis (see Fig. 3.8).

Double Palm Squeezing

Holding the palms one to six inches away from the body has a warming and tonifying effect if the giver is relaxed with their awareness centred in Tanden. This method is especially effective when applied over the face,

Off the Body Method

which can be a nice way to conclude a session. When Ki sensitivity is developed, local excess or deficiency of Ki can be clearly assessed using this technique.

Fig. 3.8: Fingers interlocked, pressure applied with heels of both hands

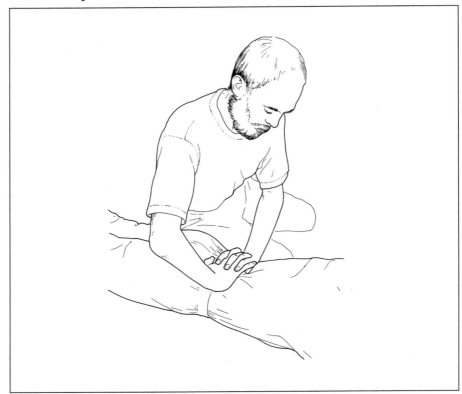

Fig. 3.9: Palms off the body

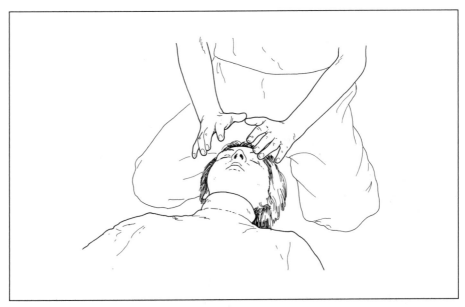

THUMBS

The thumb is a very widely used tool for Shiatsu. It is shorter and thicker than the fingers, with only one interphalangeal joint instead of two, making it the strongest individual digit. Strong pressure can therefore be applied and sustained where necessary.

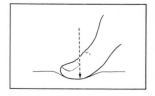

Fig. 3.10: Using ball of thumb

The ball of the thumb is used for most applications, although the area near the tip can be used when working with light pressure between small muscle groups such as in the neck.

People with stiff interphalangeal joints tend to emphasize the tip too much and are advised to adjust this, as it can be painful for the receiver. Some people have very flexible interphalangeal joints, and run the risk of overstraining them. If your thumb is of this type (see Fig. 3.12) you should use the digital ball and not the joint; and are advised to make more use of the other tools such as the palms or multiple fingers.

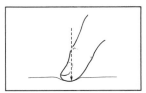

Fig. 3.11: Using area near tip

For stability it is preferable to place the other four digits lightly on the body. In an area of acute Ki distortion this allows the four fingers to remain stationary and to tonify, while the thumb actively disperses (see Fig. 3.13).

Open Hand Method

Alternatively, the four remaining digits can be formed into a fist so that the index finger can support the thumb (see Fig. 3.14). The latter is particularly useful for those with hypermobile interphalangeal joints.

Closed Hand Method

Fig. 3.12: Overstraining of interphalangeal joint

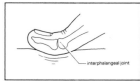

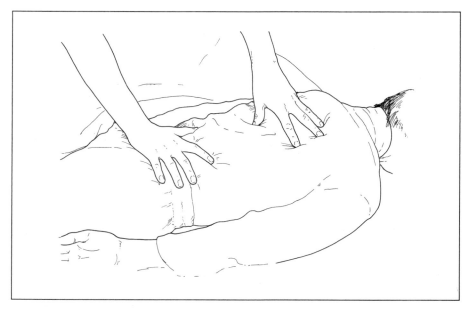

Fig. 3.13: Four fingers stationary and tonifying, thumb disperses

Fig. 3.14: Fist method

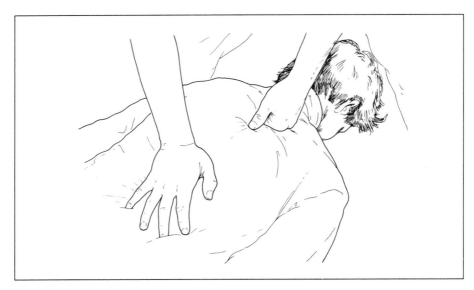

Figs 3.15(a) and (b) show other variations of thumb application which enable greater pressure to be applied to a Tsubo. However, such heavy pressure is unnecessary if treatment is accurately focused on the Kyo areas.

FINGERS

Fig. 3.15(a) Below: Thumb adjacent

Fig. 3.15(b) Below right: Thumb overlap

The fingertips are excellent tools for sensing the quality of Channel Ki because of their rich supply of sensory nerve endings. Thumbnails and fingernails should be kept short.

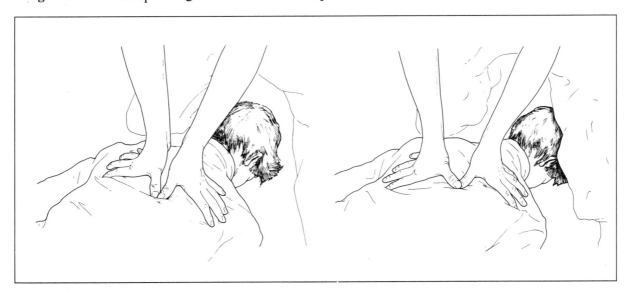

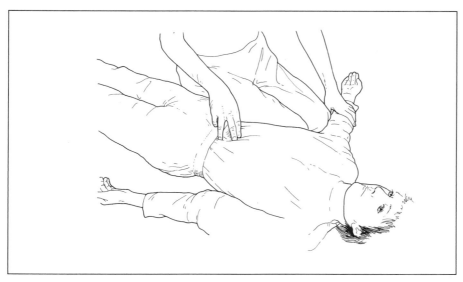

Fig. 3.16: Three fingers for Hara energy assessment

Using the second, third and fourth fingers simultaneously (i.e. the middle three) is the most versatile method. The fingers can be together or slightly apart. The thumb should be relaxed and the fingers strong (constant use of this method will quickly strengthen them). Like all Shiatsu techniques, the movement must originate from Hara, with a sense of connection to Tanden. This will give a sense of strength coming through the elbows rather than fatigue and tension accumulating in the wrist (see Fig. 3.16).

Three Finger Method

This method is used for Hara energy assessment, tracking the Channel Ki flow, and for finely tuned Ki projection and penetration.

This can be used in the same way as three fingers. A wider space between

Four Finger Method

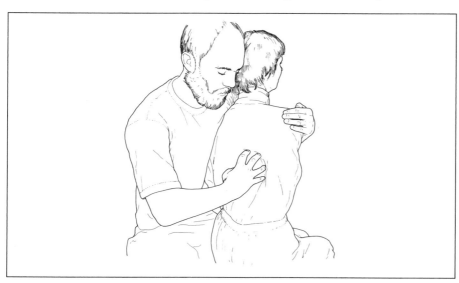

Fig. 3.17: Dispersing tension in intercostal muscles

Fig. 3.18: Pressure to side of nose

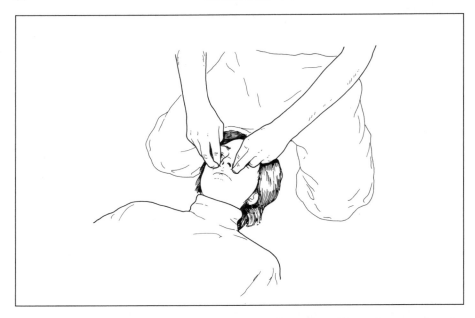

the fingers produces a configuration excellent for dispersing tension in the intercostal muscles between the ribs.

Index Finger Method   Place your middle finger on top of your index finger to give it extra support. This is a useful alternative for those with hypermobile interphalangeal thumb joints. It is very good for applying pressure to the side of the nose (see Fig. 3.18).

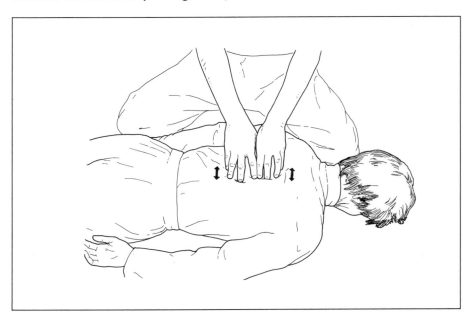

Fig. 3.19: Kenbiki

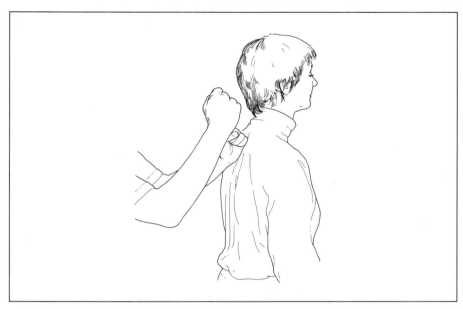

SUBSIDIARY HAND TECHNIQUES

The subsidiary hand techniques are occasionally used to disperse and calm Jitsu areas, as well as increase circulation of blood and lymph to the skin and superficial muscles. These techniques should not be applied to chronically weakened clients who have insufficient Ki, and therefore need stationary pressure to tonify their Kyo rather than dispersal techniques. (See Figs 3.19–3.25.)

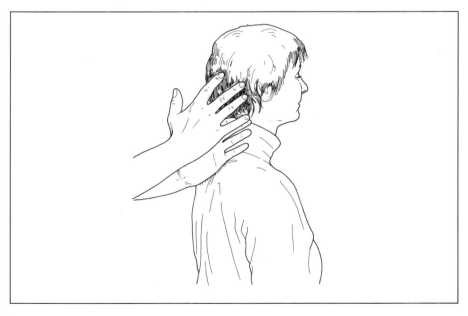

Fig. 3.21: Loose finger chopping

Fig. 3.22: Right
Cupping

Fig. 3.23: Far right
Double hand
cushioning

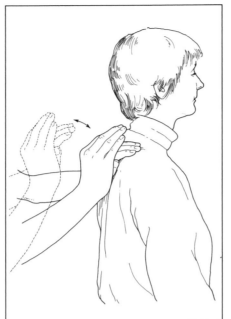 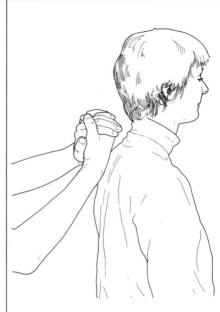

Fig. 3.24: Rocking
(very gently is OK for
Kyo recipients; more
vigorous is more
dispersing)

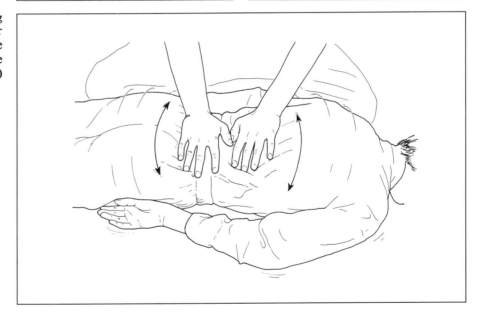

Claw Technique   Thumb and fingers are slightly curled to form a claw. The claw is then pressed into the body and quickly withdrawn as if imagining strands being pulled out of the body. In reality excess Ki is being pulled out of the area being worked on. This technique is used to disperse pockets of accumulated Ki (Jitsu areas) or stagnant Ki around the shoulder blades and buttocks, by removing it from the body completely. It is not used on the weaker client, or on Kyo areas. (See Fig. 3.26.)

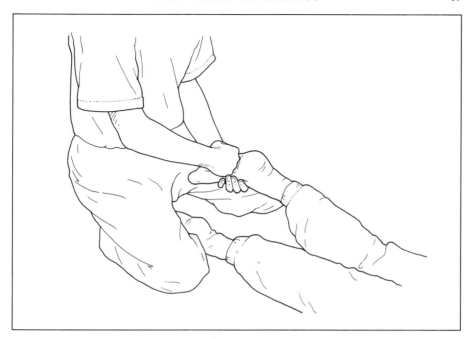

Fig. 3.25: Knuckle rolling (on the feet)

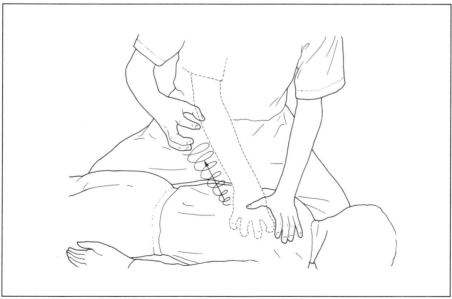

Fig. 3.26: Ki being pulled out of the body

The middle and index fingers are pressed simultaneously either side of the spinal column in small infants, or in the intercostal spaces close to either side of the sternum in adults.

'Vee' Finger Technique

The thumb and index finger are spread wide. Pressure is applied through the wide angle 'vee' shape, with pressure falling mainly on the

'Dragon's Mouth' Technique

Fig. 3.27: Dragon's
Mouth to occiput

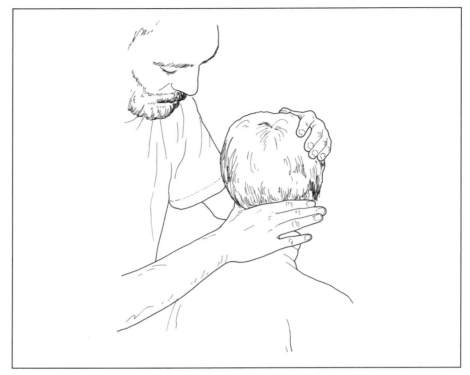

Fig. 3.28: Dragon's
Mouth with both
hands to waistline

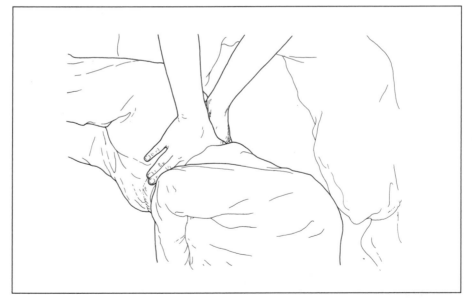

proximal joint of the index finger. The 'Dragon's mouth' can be used to
apply pressure just above the knee or to the occiput. Both hands can be
placed together to apply pressure to the waist in the sidelying position
(see Figs 3.27, 3.28).

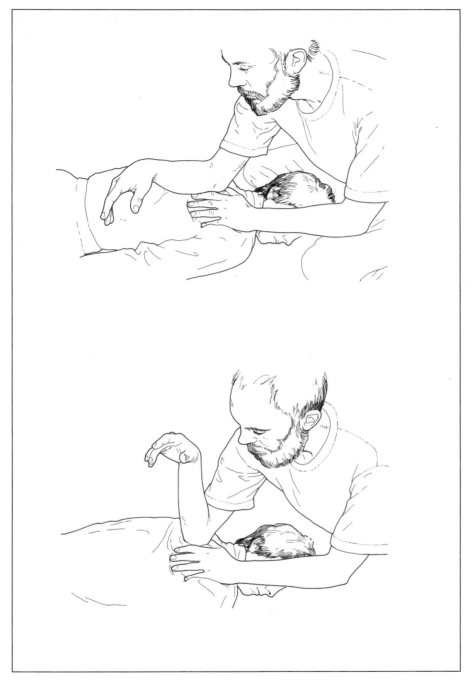

Fig. 3.29: Variety of elbow joint angles

ELBOWS

The elbows, or the area of forearm close to the elbows, can be used to apply strong pressure to the back, hips and feet. They should be used with care, and applied only to areas which have already been palpated by the hands. This is because they are far less sensitive than the hands.

An acutely flexed elbow joint gives the strongest pressure, which in most cases is too much. A more open elbow joint gives a more comfortable pressure, which can be varied according to the angle of the elbow joint. It is essential to keep the wrist relaxed and fist open. (See Fig. 3.29.)

The elbow should not be used before a high level of sensitivity has developed in the hands. Premature use of elbow techniques will reduce the number of friends willing to receive your Shiatsu!

KNEES

The knees can give very firm pressure, so should be used with discretion only to areas previously checked by the hands. They can be applied individually or both together, but the majority of your body weight should be kept back on your haunches, or equally distributed through the hands.

Maximum support should be given so that the knees can be instantly removed if necessary to ensure the receiver's comfort and your own stability. (See Fig. 3.30.)

FEET

Feet can be used as a tool for Shiatsu, and although they are less sensitive than the hands, they can give a very 'earthy' ingredient to a

Fig 3.30: Knees on inner thighs in sidelying

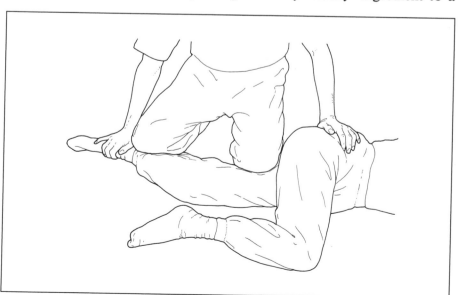

session. This is perhaps because they spend most of their time in contact with the ground. If you intend to use your feet you should walk around in bare feet as much as possible to give them an even greater earthy quality.

Using the feet gives you a chance to stand up if you have been giving Shiatsu with your hands for several hours. They can be used to tonify the ankles, which in turn helps to tonify the kidneys (see Fig 3.31). Generally however, they are more useful for temporarily dispersing Jitsu areas in the limbs by using a rapid shaking technique, but with light pressure (see Fig 3.32). This may be useful for dispersing excessive

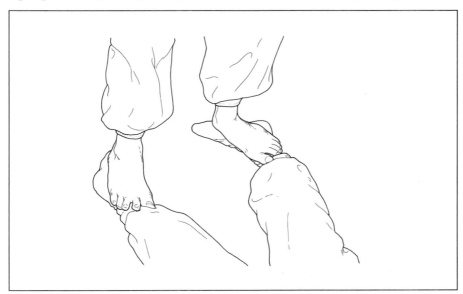

Fig. 3.31: Standing on ankles to tonify the kidneys . . . but only if ankles are flexible enough

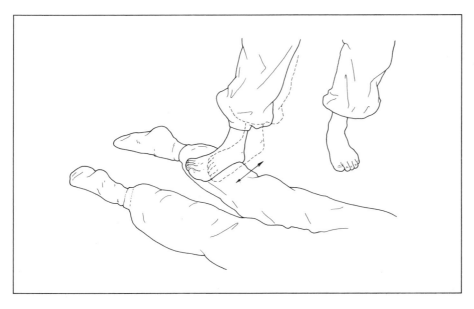

Fig. 3.32: Vigorous shaking of foot on calf muscles – *avoid knee joint*

surface tension when it is masking underlying Kyo, thus rendering the Kyo more accessible to hand palpation.

Feet are useful tools to anchor the recipient's body when certain stretches are applied (see Fig. 3.33).

Fig. 3.33: Body anchored in prone lying, leg stretched

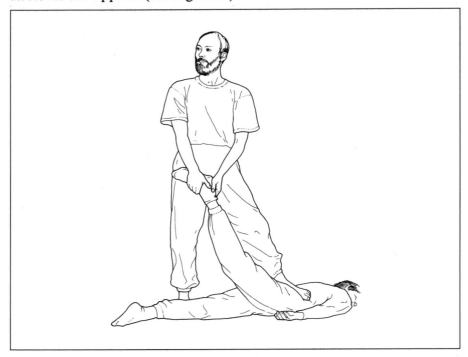

To apply Shiatsu using the feet requires that you keep your centre of gravity as low as possible by constantly imagining the feet are being filled from Tanden with sand or some other heavy substance.

BREATHING

The correct way to breathe for both the giver and receiver comes automatically provided both are relaxed. The level of relaxation in the receiver is largely influenced by the degree of relaxation in the giver, due to the close proximity and energy-based nature of Shiatsu.

When pressure or stretch is applied, it is natural for both giver and receiver to gently exhale. Inhalation naturally takes place when pressure is released. The more relaxed you are, the longer will be the period of no-breathing between exhalation and inhalation. The no-breathing phase is when there is maximum receptivity to subtle changes in muscle tone or Ki flow. However, it is quite common to discover that your recipient simply cannot fully relax because they are not in touch with their breathing. For these people it is helpful to tell them to consciously breathe out as you apply pressure. After several repetitions of dictated

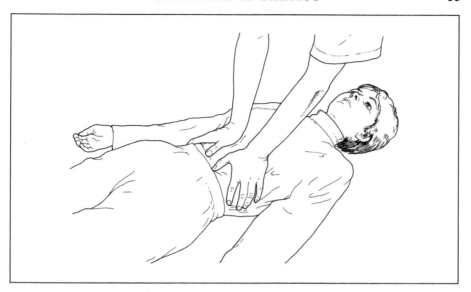

Fig. 3.34:
Mechanically assisting exhalation using palm pressure on the ribs, in supine

breathing, they usually make the correction and all is well. In some cases it is helpful to apply pressure to their lower ribs as you tell them to exhale, thus giving their lungs some mechanical assistance (see Fig 3.34).

Chapter 4

Shiatsu Channel Outlines

Some styles of Shiatsu use no Channels at all, some use the traditional acupuncture Channels, while others use the extended Channel system expounded by Shizuto Masunaga. For family orientated Shiatsu it is not necessary to use the Channels to achieve basic relaxation and to alleviate minor aches and pains. However, even with family orientated Shiatsu, one begins to feel specific differences between different areas within a given space, such as say, the thigh. If Ki sensitivity is consciously being developed through the diligent practice of Shiatsu – and perhaps reinforced through Aikido or Qi Gong – and if the mind of the exponent is curious enough, the Channels begin to present themselves. Having said that, it would take a long time to recognize them spontaneously for what they are, and what they represent. Hence we give you a map.

The Classical Channels present a grid for the location and treatment of fixed Tsubos. However, tactile experience reveals that each Channel can be strongly influenced by Shiatsu applied to certain other areas of the body. These areas or 'extensions' are most clearly represented in the limbs. Each of the six Classical Channels in the arms have corresponding energy extensions in the legs. Likewise, the six leg Channels have related extensions in the arms. These extensions sometimes follow the course of another Channel. For example, the Heart Channel's extension at the postero-medial aspect of the thigh lies over the Classical Kidney Channel.

Since no fixed Tsubos appear on the extensions, they are of little value to acupuncturists. However, since the Channels are affected by the penetration of touch into the extensions, they prove invaluable to the Shiatsu therapist.

This idea of Channel extension was first put forward by Shizuto Masunaga, who was primarily responsible for promoting their use.

Both the Classical Channels and their extended Channel pathways are presented as a map on the following pages.

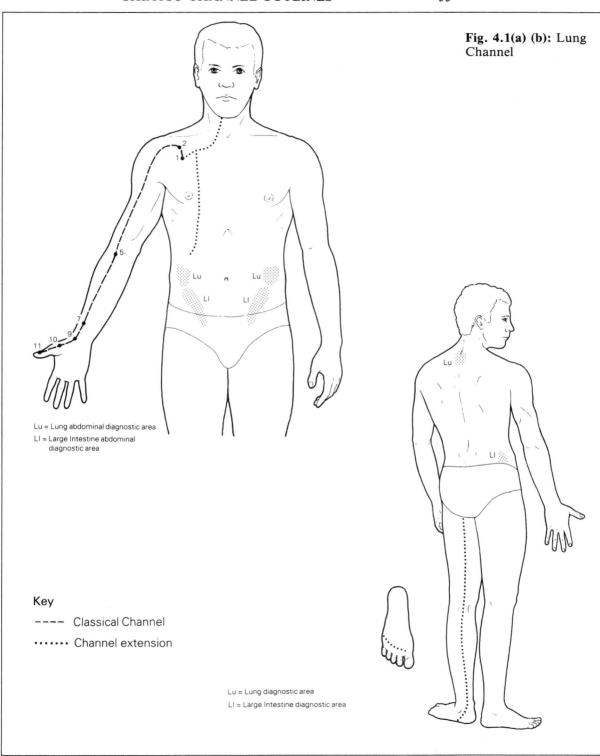

Fig. 4.1(a) (b): Lung Channel

Lu = Lung abdominal diagnostic area

Ll = Large Intestine abdominal
       diagnostic area

Key

---- Classical Channel

.... Channel extension

Lu = Lung diagnostic area

Ll = Large Intestine diagnostic area

Fig. 4.2(a) (b): Large
Intestine Channel

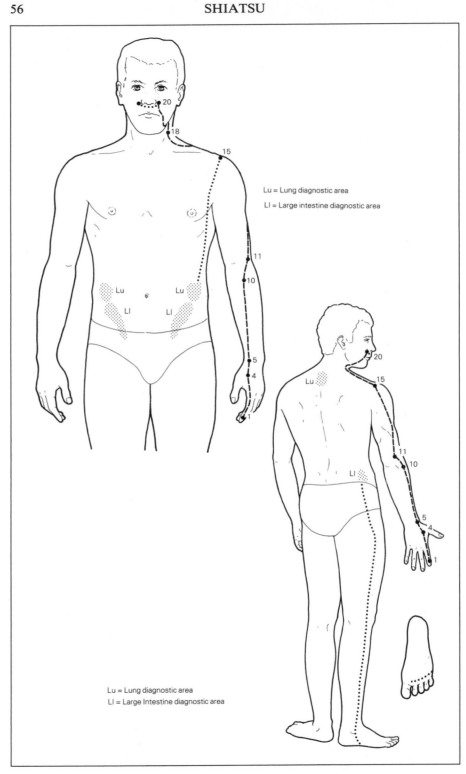

Lu = Lung diagnostic area

LI = Large intestine diagnostic area

Lu = Lung diagnostic area
LI = Large Intestine diagnostic area

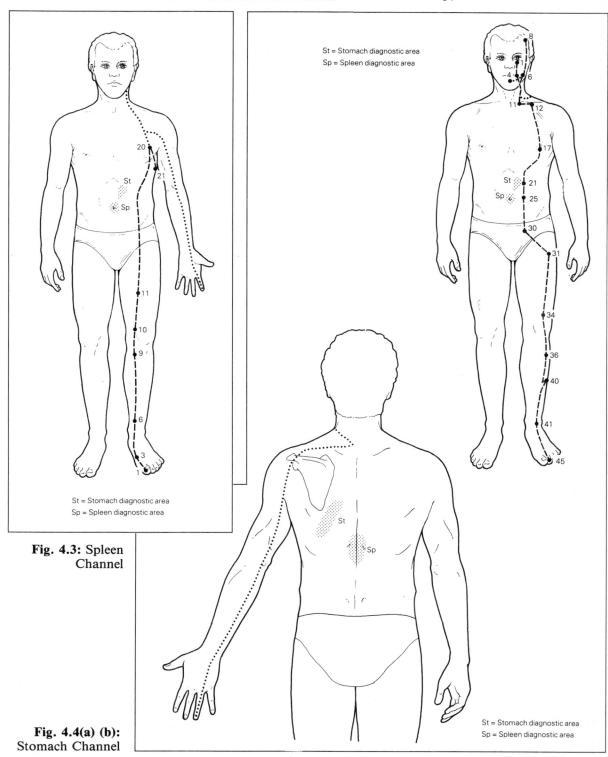

St = Stomach diagnostic area
Sp = Spleen diagnostic area

St = Stomach diagnostic area
Sp = Spleen diagnostic area

St = Stomach diagnostic area
Sp = Spleen diagnostic area

Fig. 4.3: Spleen
Channel

Fig. 4.4(a) (b):
Stomach Channel

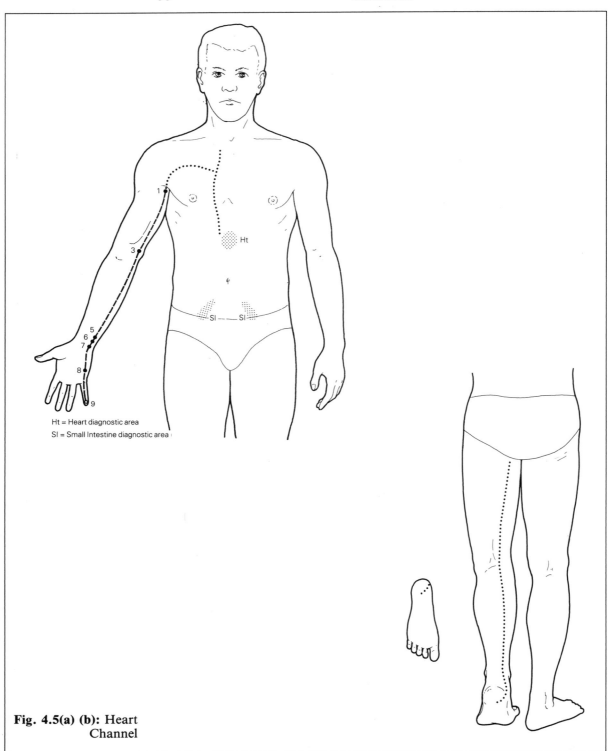

Ht = Heart diagnostic area
SI = Small Intestine diagnostic area

Fig. 4.5(a) (b): Heart
Channel

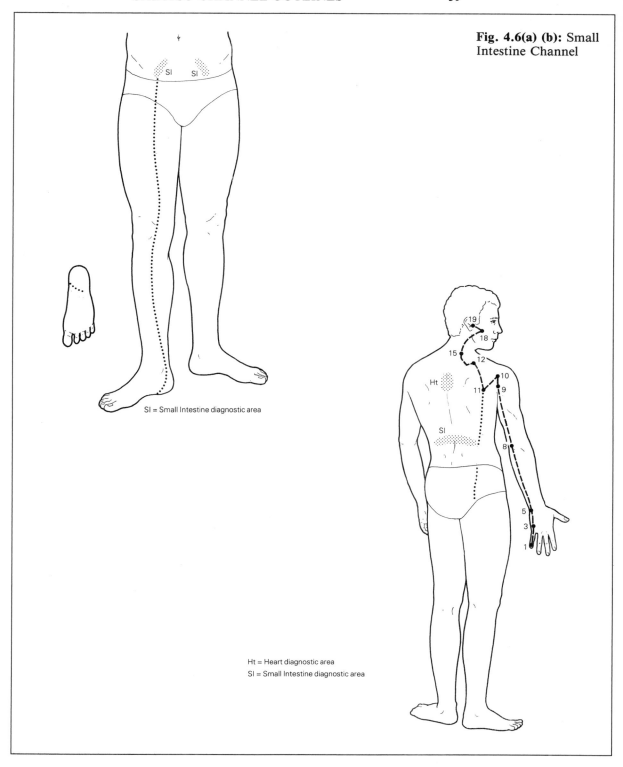

Fig. 4.6(a) (b): Small Intestine Channel

SI = Small Intestine diagnostic area

Ht = Heart diagnostic area
SI = Small Intestine diagnostic area

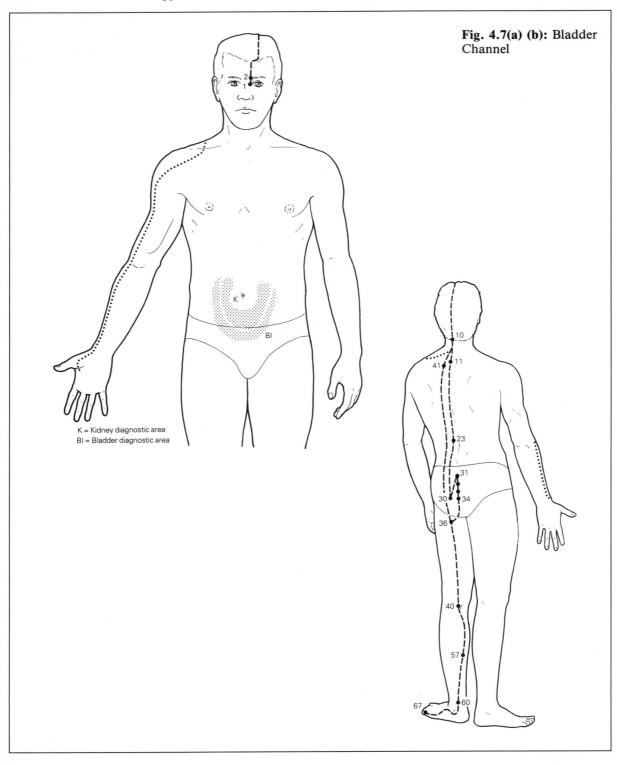

Fig. 4.7(a) (b): Bladder Channel

K = Kidney diagnostic area
Bl = Bladder diagnostic area

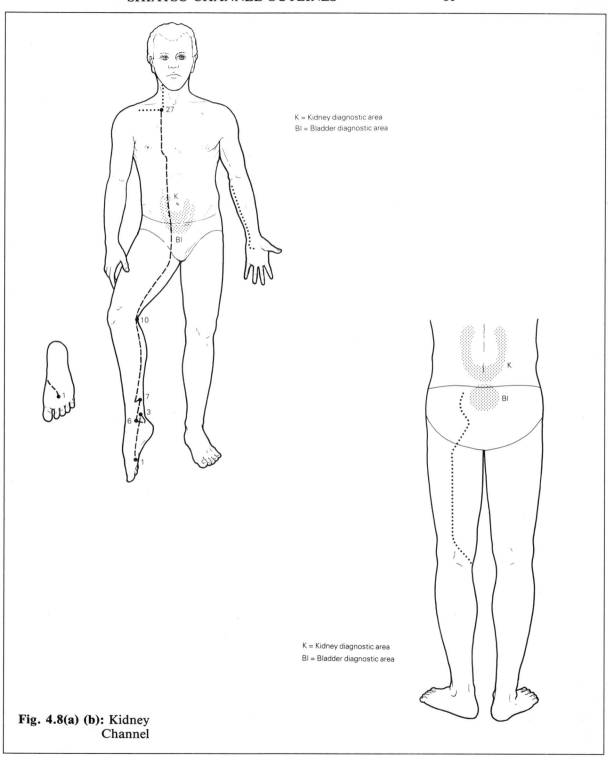

K = Kidney diagnostic area
Bl = Bladder diagnostic area

K = Kidney diagnostic area
Bl = Bladder diagnostic area

Fig. 4.8(a) (b): Kidney Channel

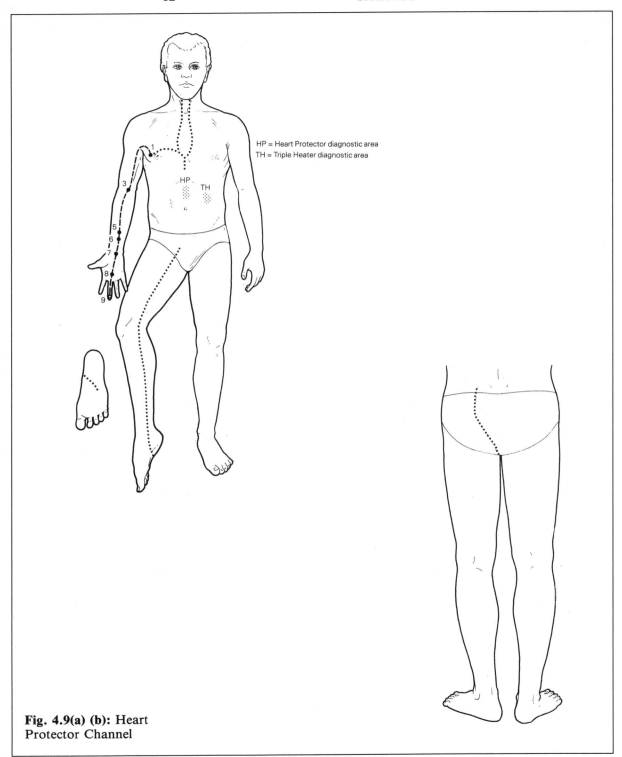

HP = Heart Protector diagnostic area
TH = Triple Heater diagnostic area

Fig. 4.9(a) (b): Heart
Protector Channel

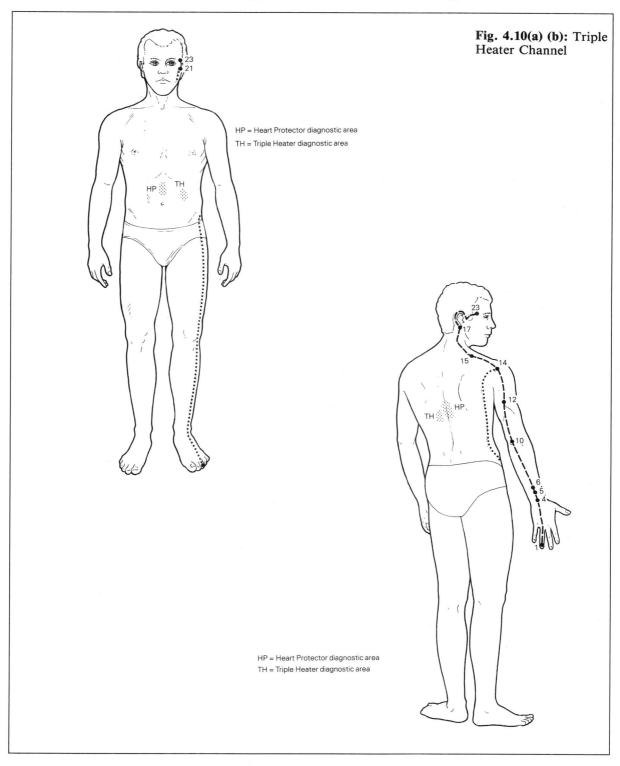

Fig. 4.10(a) (b): Triple Heater Channel

HP = Heart Protector diagnostic area
TH = Triple Heater diagnostic area

HP = Heart Protector diagnostic area
TH = Triple Heater diagnostic area

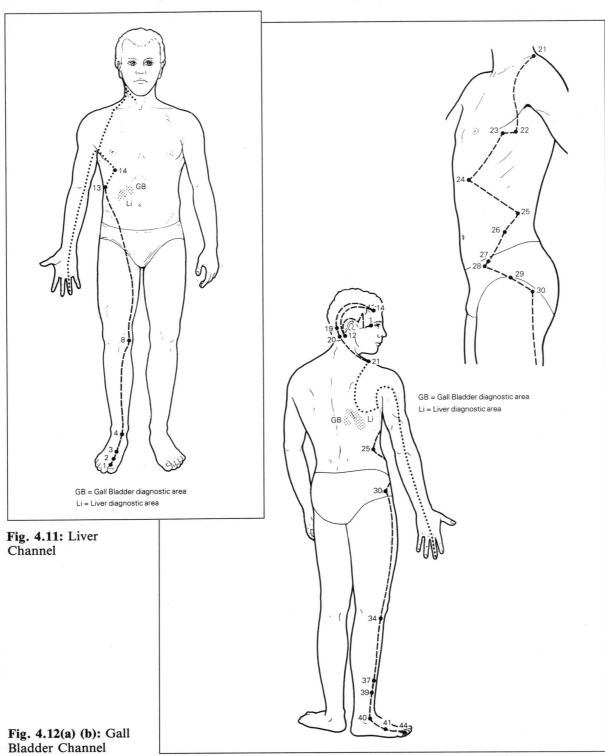

GB = Gall Bladder diagnostic area
Li = Liver diagnostic area

Fig. 4.11: Liver Channel

GB = Gall Bladder diagnostic area
Li = Liver diagnostic area

Fig. 4.12(a) (b): Gall Bladder Channel

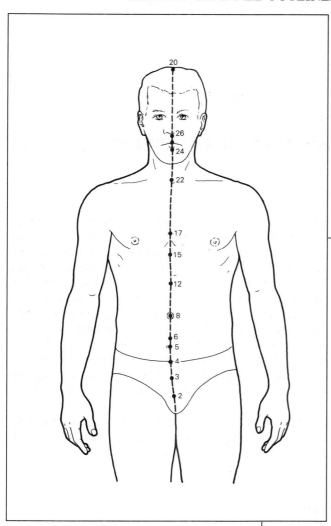

Fig. 4.13: Directing
Vessel Channel

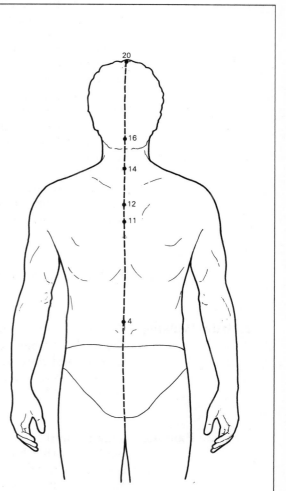

Fig. 4.14: Governing
Vessel Channel

Chapter 5

Basic Shiatsu Technique

This chapter will present a variety of techniques for each main position in which the receiver can be placed, namely, face down, face up, sidelying and sitting, giving an overall general sequence which is by no means exhaustive, as the possibilities for technique variation are endless. You should bear in mind that each of us are of unique physical proportions so that all of these techniques will suit some people, and some techniques will suit all people. Most of us however, will be inclined to abandon certain techniques and make slight adaptations to others. This adds to the creativity of Shiatsu, which is important if a flexible reaction to the infinite variety of interrelationships between giver and receiver is to be maintained. Please adapt, adjust and accommodate without sacrificing any of the essential elements of Shiatsu outlined in Chapter 2.

If you are the type of person who prefers to work with a well defined structure, then these sequences can provide a basic framework into which you can add the stretches described in Chapter 6.

FACE DOWN POSITION

1. Baby Walking This technique is so named because the giver should simply walk over the receiver's back and buttocks using the palms, with the same lack of tension and natural use of body weight as a baby would do. Keep the palms relaxed and avoid the spinal column. This technique is comforting for the receiver and helps the giver 'connect' (see Fig. 5.1).

2. Palming This is similar to baby walking except you keep one hand stationary while the other hand explores the back. Consciousness should be in the stationary hand to feel for any changes in muscle tone or movement of Ki, and to maintain a sense of connection between the two hands. This technique is more effective if the support hand is connected to a particularly Kyo area.

One hand on the scapula, the other hand on the buttocks. Repeat crossing arms and also try using forearms instead of hands (see Fig. 5.2).

3. Diagonal Stretch

Rock from your Hara rather than just from your hands. Find the receiver's natural rocking rhythm and go with it. Gently is very calming; more vigorous is dispersing (see Fig. 5.3).

4. Rocking

Move the skin and connective tissues over the sacral bone rather than friction rub the surface. This technique stimulates circulation to the pelvic region and can move Ki that has stagnated there, but should be avoided if the Bladder Channel is Kyo (see Fig. 5.4).

5. Sacral Rub

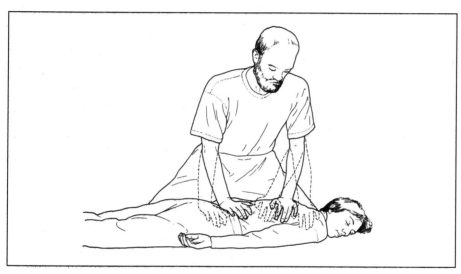

Fig. 5.1: Baby walking: relaxed body; weight underside; maximum connection

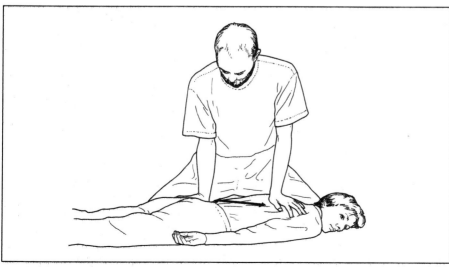

Fig. 5.2: Diagonal stretch

Fig. 5.3: Rocking

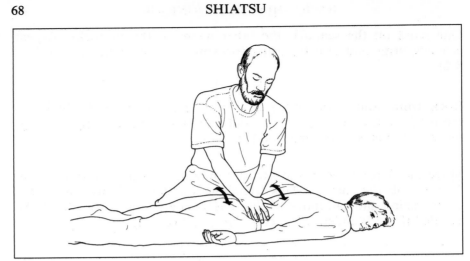

Fig. 5.4: Sacral rub

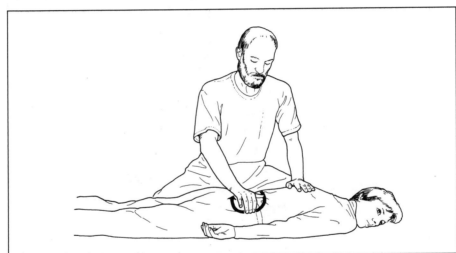

Fig. 5.5: Retreating cat

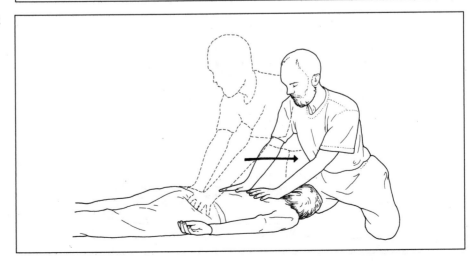

Walking hands from buttocks to shoulders and down arms. This will prepare Bladder Channel for subsequent thumb pressure technique (see Fig. 5.5).

6. 'Retreating Cat'

7. Thumb Down Bladder Channel

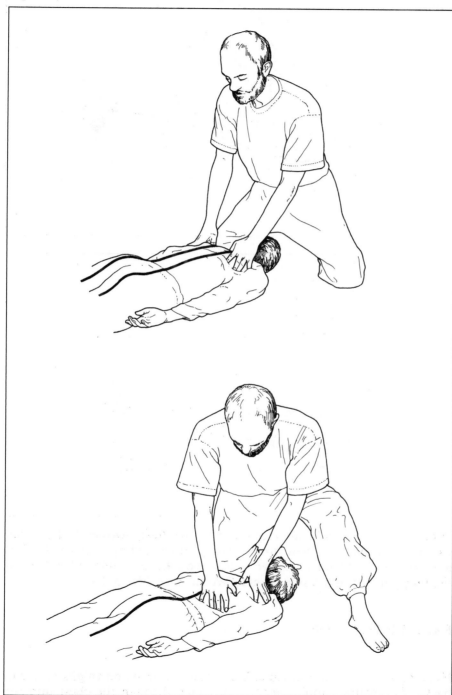

Fig. 5.6(a): Above
Thumb down Bladder Channel – 2 thumb technique

Fig. 5.6(b): Left
Thumb down Bladder Channel – 1 thumb technique with support hand

8. Working on Bladder Channel in Legs

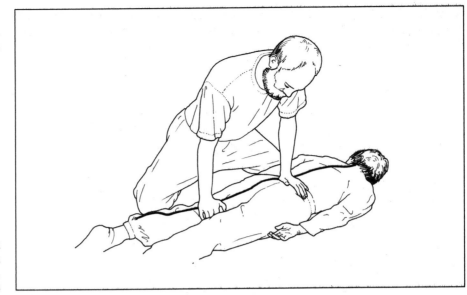

Fig. 5.7: Working on Bladder Channel in legs. First use palms, then use thumbs

Fig. 5.8: Forearm into sole of foot

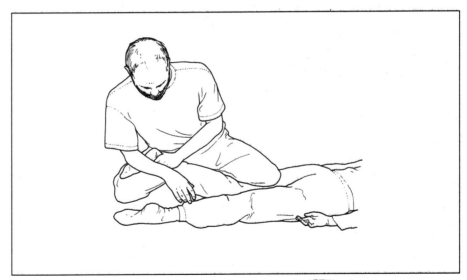

9. Forearms into Sole of Foot Support hand clasps firmly around ankle, to tonify Kidney and Bladder Channels. Make sure their instep is fully supported by your thigh. This may be uncomfortable for you until you have developed sufficient flexibility in toe and ankle plantarflexion. (See Fig. 5.8.)

FACE UP POSITION

1. Pulling Heels Hold heels rather than grasp ankles. Rest forearms on thighs and lean back. The feeling should be of lengthening through the chest into the

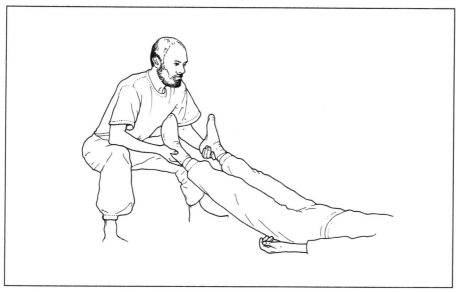

Fig. 5.9: Pulling heels

Fig. 5.10(a): Below left
Knee to chest

back of the head. Shaking from side to side with a gentle 'whip-like' action is also useful from this position as a general loosener.

Fig. 5.10(b): Below
Knee to chest

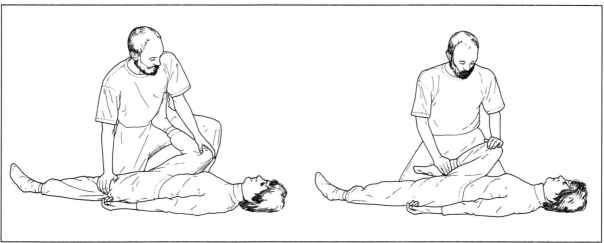

Two variations illustrated (Fig. 5.10 a and b). This technique mildly lengthens the lumbar and gluteal musculature.

2. Knee to Chest

It is very supportive to keep your body in full contact with the recipient's leg (see Fig. 5.11).

3. Hip Rotations

Hold their foot 'protectively' into your Hara and gently rotate your whole body. This is incredibly supportive, nurturing and 'grounding' for the receiver and one of the most centring and relaxing techniques to give. The other leg can be worked on in the same way.

4. Baby-Rocking the Foot

Fig. 5.11: Hip rotation

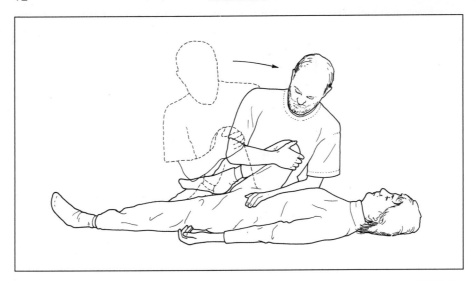

Fig. 5.12: Baby-rocking the foot

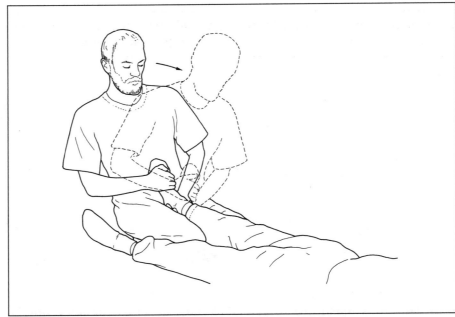

5. Hand to Hara   This is a comforting way to relax the receiver while tonifying the Heart Channel. It is very centring to give. Use palm first, then thumb on upper arm, fingertips on forearm (see Fig. 5.13).

Finger Tip Occiput Support   This is excellent for tonifying the Gall Bladder Channel if it is Kyo in the occipital area. Fingertips are contacting GB20 and can connect with all

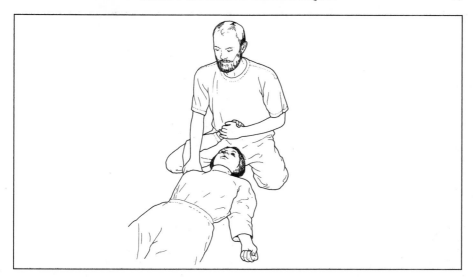

Fig. 5.13: Hand to Hara

the occipital points (BL 10 and GV 16). Avoid working directly on the occiput if this area is Jitsu, because it could bring on a headache.

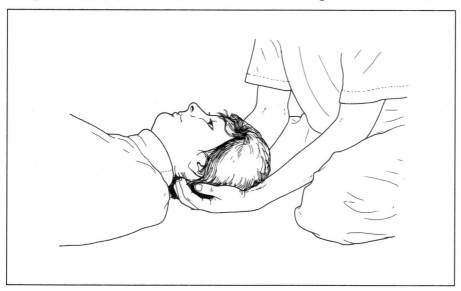

Fig. 5.14: Finger tip occiput support

SIDELYING POSITION

Rotate the shoulder with receiver's forearm resting over yours, keeping maximum body contact and moving your whole body from your Hara. This enables the recipient to relax into it better (see Fig. 5.15).

1. Shoulder Girdle Rotation

Forearm connects to front of shoulder. Lean weight through both hands simultaneously (see Fig. 5.16).

2. Head Press

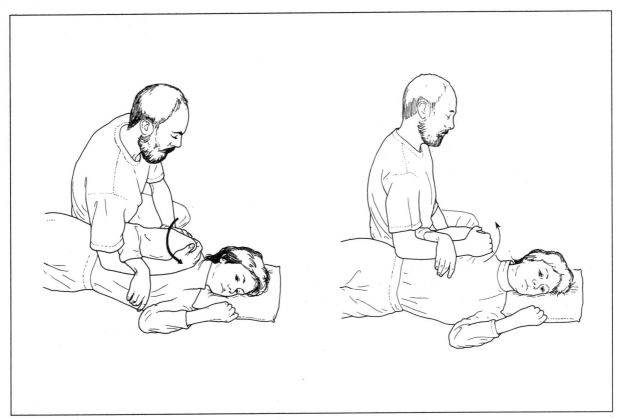

Fig. 5.15: Shoulder girdle rotation

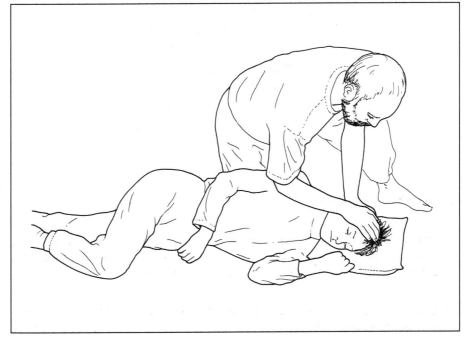

Fig. 5.16: Head press

Support hand rests diagonally opposite occiput, near forehead. Forearms connect to front of shoulder. Thumbs or fingertips connect into occipital Tsubos including GB 20, BL 10 and GV 16, and then into neck from occiput to nape of neck (see Fig. 5.17).

3. Occipital Opening/Neck Release

Use fingertips or heel of hand to disperse Jitsu in Small Intestine, Gall Bladder or Triple Heater Channels in the scapula area (see Fig. 5.18).

4. Shoulder Girdle Dispersing Technique

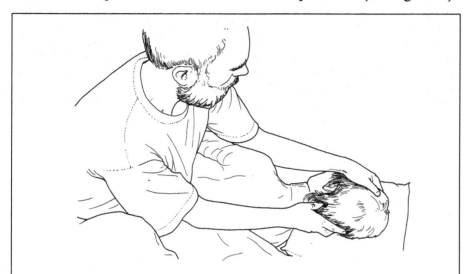

Fig. 5.17: Occipital opening/neck release

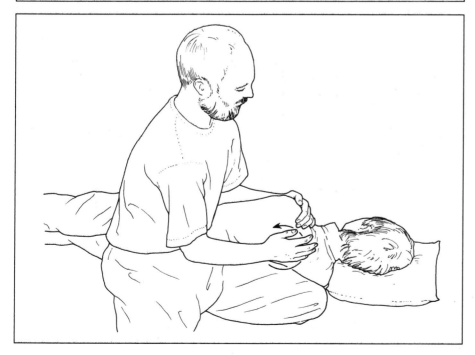

Fig. 5.18: Shoulder girdle dispersing technique

5. Scapula Loosening   Scapula is folded over fingertips. Working hand is supported by the thigh. Difficulty getting under one side only can indicate postural imbalance such as scoliosis. Right scapula stiffness may indicate a congested liver. Left scapula stiffness may indicate acid Stomach. Stiffness in both may be due to Liver congestion; therefore this technique is a useful aid in decongesting the Liver (see Fig. 5.19).

6. Knees Into Back   Use palms initially to feel whether or not knee pressure is appropriate. One knee tonifies a Kyo area, while the other knee disperses Jitsu areas. Good hand support on shoulder and hip is essential. Strong Shiatsu can be given to the Bladder, Kidney and Small Intestine Channels using this technique. Please ensure that stationary pressure is applied perpendicular to the surface of the body (see Fig. 5.20).

     This technique can be applied around the sacro-iliac and hip joints.

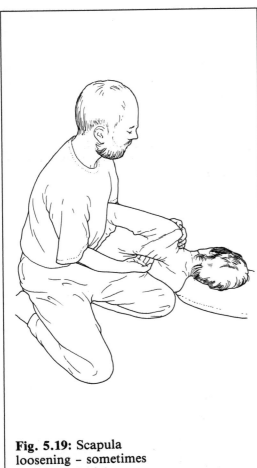

Fig. 5.19: Scapula loosening – sometimes called the 'chicken wing'

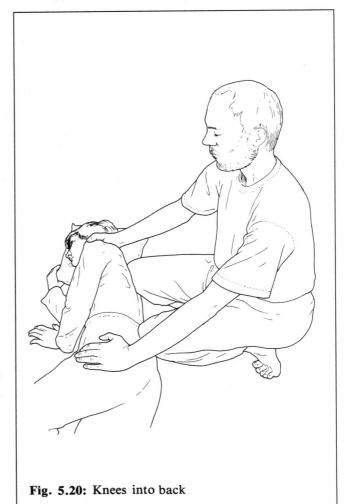

Fig. 5.20: Knees into back

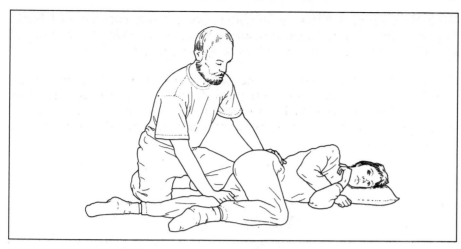

7. Palms/Knees into Heart Channel extension

Fig. 5.21: Palms/knees into Heart Channel

SITTING POSITION

All these techniques could be done with the receiver sitting in a chair or sitting with legs outstretched, although more support will be required.

Apply two-handed pressure in a variety of positions across lower back and upper buttocks.

1. Child's Pose

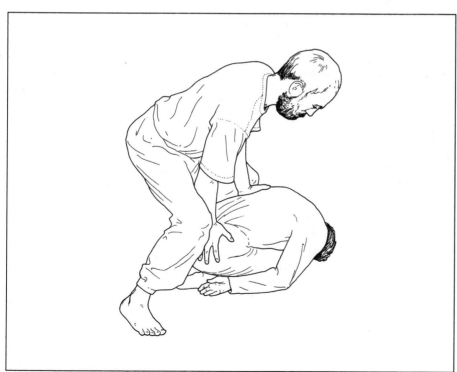

Fig. 5.22: Child's pose

2. Palming the Back   With firm support hand on shoulder, palm down each side of back. Support hand should be on the same side as the working hand, i.e. left shoulder supported, left side of back worked (see Fig. 5.23).

3. Neck Rotations   The neck should be rotated in a posterior semi-circle and never through a full circle, which can damage the facet joints of the cervical vertebrae.

Neck rotations done well can relieve tension in the neck muscles and move Ki stagnation in the occiput, especially around BL-10 and GB-20 (see Fig. 5.24).

Fig. 5.23: Palming the back

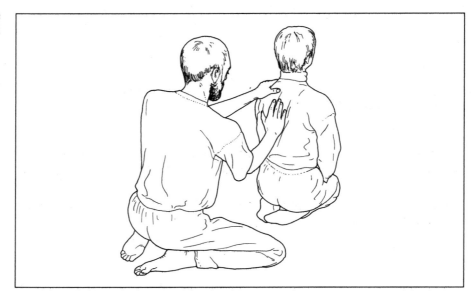

Fig. 5.24: Neck rotations

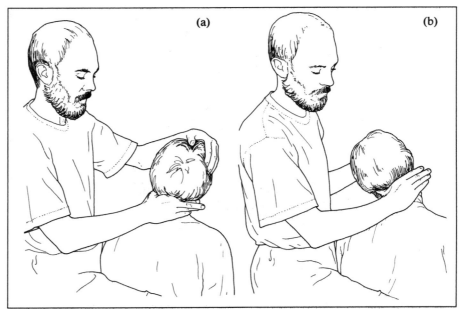

Large Intestine Channel can be given maximum support in the arm and shoulder with this technique (see Fig. 5.25).

4. Forearm into Trapezius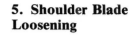

Shoulder blades are folded back over fingertips. Inability to get under the shoulder blades can indicate GB Kyo or Jitsu: liver congestion on the right side, Stomach acidity on the left side (see Fig. 5.26).

5. Shoulder Blade Loosening

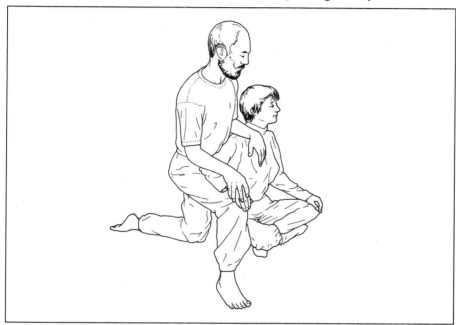

Fig. 5.25: Forearm into trapezius

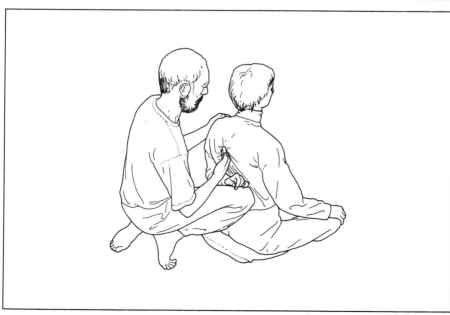

Fig. 5.26: Scapula loosening

SHIATSU TO THE HARA AND CHEST

The Hara and Chest are very sensitive and protected parts of the body, and as such the receiver's confidence must be gained before Shiatsu can be administered there. However, under circumstances of mutual trust they can be extremely effective areas to work.

Generally the giver should be positioned on the right side of the receiver because many of the techniques, if done from this side, will facilitate the peristaltic movement of the bowel, particularly in the transverse colon where the bowel movement travels from right to left. Wave rocking is a good example of this.

1. Wave Rocking   Kneeling, facing Hara. One hand on top of the other, knead the belly with a motion similar to a wave breaking upon the shore. This is good for moving Ki, and so should not be done on a very Kyo Hara (see Fig. 5.27).

2. Bowl Rotations   Form an inverted bowl with both hands. Rotate the bowl's rim around client's belly, upon a central axis, in a clockwise direction (see Fig. 5.28).

3. Bowl Circling   As above, for 2, but circle the axis of the bowl over the client's belly in a clockwise direction, thereby stretching the fascia more. This is excellent for sluggish bowels and poor abdominal circulation, but not suitable for very Kyo conditions (see Fig. 5.29).

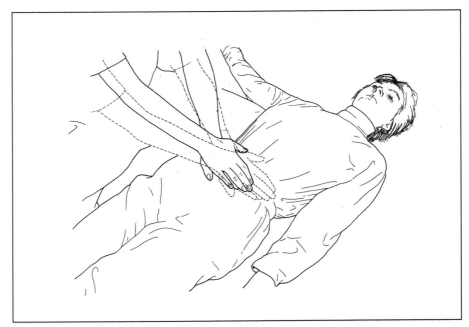

Fig. 5.27: Wave rocking

The previous three techniques can also be done with one hand on the Hara, while the other gives support under the lumbar spine.

Gather the belly flesh to centre with both hands, from varying directions, but generally progressing in a clockwise direction (see Fig. 5.30).

4. Gathering to 'Centre'

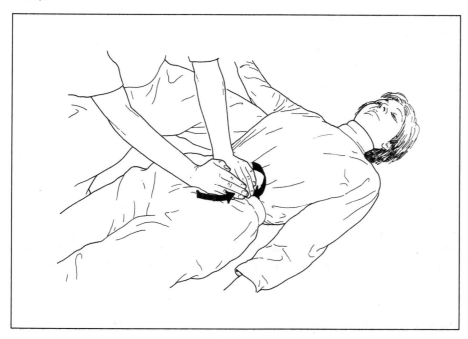

Fig. 5.28: Bowl rotations

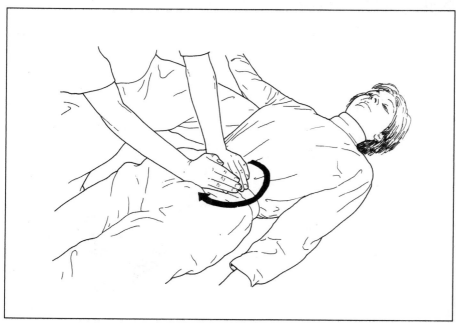

Fig. 5.29: Bowl circling

Fig. 5.30: Gathering to
centre

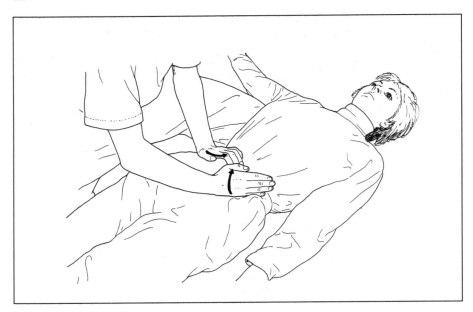

All the previous techniques tend to disperse Jitsu. To tonify Kyo it is effective to simply hold perpendicular, stationary, focused touch, with palms or fingertips, provided there is a strong support hand nearby.

5. Sternal Cupping   Place edges of both hands on either side of the sternum and lean in gently as receiver exhales (see Fig. 5.31).

Fig. 5.31: Sternal
cupping

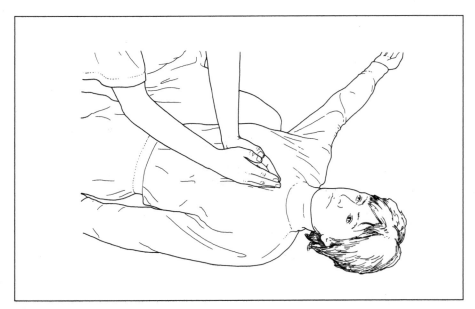

Chapter 6

Stretching

Stretching is a useful component of Shiatsu because it can:

- Improve flexibility
- Improve blood and lymphatic circulation
- Bring Channels closer to the surface
- Help disperse sections of a Channel and ease muscular tension
- Improve respiration by opening the rib cage

However, to apply stretch effectively, certain principles must be understood. A muscle consists of numerous contractile fibres bound together in parallel groups encased within a sheath of connective tissue. The sheath extends beyond the muscle fibres to form a strong fibrous cord known as a tendon, which attaches the muscle to the bone.

At rest, all muscles remain in a state of slight contraction called *tonus*. On receiving an impulse from a motor nerve, the muscle will contract further and shorten in length. On cessation of that impulse it will cease to shorten and return to a state of tonus.

Muscles usually work in pairs; for example the biceps muscle flexes the elbow and the triceps muscle extends the elbow. To allow the biceps to shorten and flex the elbow, the triceps must reduce its level of contraction, otherwise they would fight against each other and prevent movement from occurring. The muscle contracting to produce a movement is referred to as the *agonist* or *prime mover*, whereas the opposite muscle which relaxes to allow the movement is known as the *antagonist*. The degree of relaxation and lengthening in the antagonist is proportional to the strength and extent of contraction by the agonist. Therefore the more strongly the biceps contracts against resistance to flex the elbow joint, the more the triceps can relax and lengthen. Other muscles which increase in tonus to stabilize the rest of the body and prevent other joints from moving during agonist/antagonist interplay are known as *synergists* or *fixators*.

A muscle cannot be stretched as such because its fibres are not elastic, but actively contractile. Therefore the way to lengthen a muscle to achieve a greater range of movement is to reduce its tonus. This can be achieved by persuading the muscle's protective mechanisms to co-operate, which requires an understanding of the stretch reflex.

Fig. 6.1:
Muscle/tendon
structure

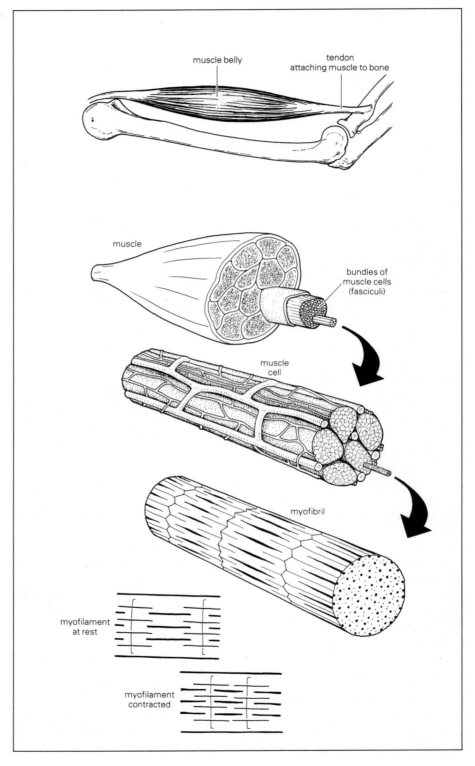

muscle belly

tendon attaching muscle to bone

muscle

bundles of muscle cells (fasciculi)

muscle cell

myofibril

myofilament at rest

myofilament contracted

THE STRETCH REFLEX

Nerves known as *muscle spindles* are connected in parallel to various muscle cells at intervals throughout the muscle. When the muscle lengthens, so do the muscle spindles. If the muscle is lengthened too quickly and too much, the muscle spindle will react by sending an impulse via the spinal cord telling the muscle to contract. This is a protective mechanism to prevent injury resulting from sudden overstretching, and is known as the stretch reflex.

When a person falls asleep in a sitting position, the head will relax forward, then jerk back up. This is an example of muscle spindle reflex within the muscles at the back of the neck (see Fig. 6.2).

Although the muscle spindle responds when the muscle is stretched unexpectedly, it does permit voluntary lengthening if it is slow and gradual.

Other nerve cells called tendon organs exist where the tendons join the muscle fibres. When the muscle is strongly contracted, the tendon organs are stretched, which initiates an impulse to the muscle telling it to relax. This is therefore the opposite of the stretch reflex insofar as muscle spindles cause muscles to contract when they are overstretched, whereas tendon organs relax muscles when they are overcontracted.

A muscle can be made to lengthen further than usual by first strongly contracting it to initiate a relaxation response from the tendon organs, and then lengthening the muscle slowly to avoid stimulating the muscle spindles (see Fig. 6.3).

This type of muscle lengthening is called *facilitated stretching* (or proprioceptive neuromuscular facilitation: PNF) and is the most effective way to increase flexibility. It is a major ingredient of the corrective exercise system known as Sotai.

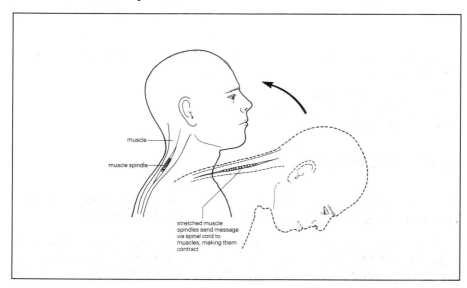

muscle

muscle spindle

stretched muscle spindles send message via spinal cord to muscles, making them contract

Fig. 6.2: Muscle spindles sending message to muscles at back of neck via spinal cord

Fig. 6.3(a): Prone lying: front thigh muscles contracted strongly against resistance showing tendon organs relaying messages to 'relax' via spinal cord

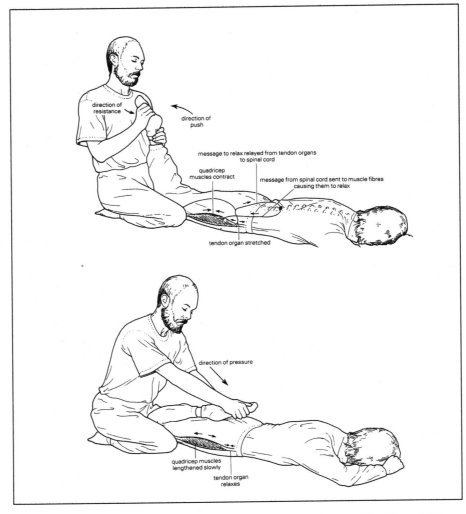

direction of resistance

direction of push

message to relax relayed from tendon organs to spinal cord

quadricep muscles contract

message from spinal cord sent to muscle fibres causing them to relax

tendon organ stretched

direction of pressure

quadricep muscles lengthened slowly

tendon organ relaxes

Fig. 6.3(b): Lengthen muscle slowly to avoid stimulating muscle spindles

There are three methods of lengthening muscles applicable within a Shiatsu session:

- Gravity stretching
- Passive assisted stretching
- Facilitated stretching

GRAVITY STRETCHING

Maximum support is given to anchor the body so that a specific muscle group can lengthen by surrendering to gravity (see Fig. 6.4).

With gravity stretching, the muscle spindle might initiate a muscle tonus for a few seconds, but the sustained opening of the muscle will pacify the spindles' impulses and allow more lengthening within two

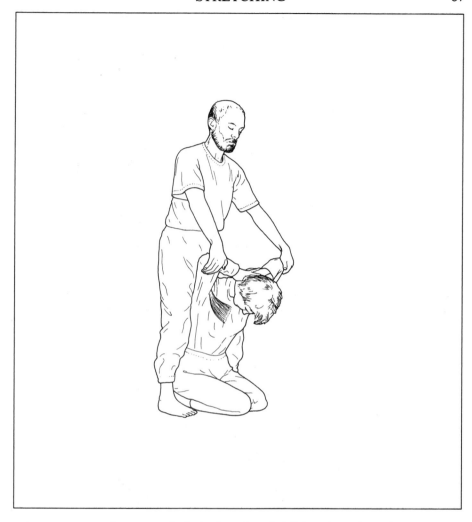

Fig. 6.4: Gravity stretch – lengthening pectoral muscles. In kneeling, elbows supported, client relaxes forward; gravity acts on body weight to lengthen pectoral muscles

minutes, assuming no pain is induced to inhibit relaxation. Slow, deep, rhythmical breathing helps.

PASSIVE ASSISTED STRETCHING

With passive assisted stretching the muscle being lengthened is very gently coaxed further with the help of a partner. This method operates by the same principle as gravity stretching, but is more effective (see Fig. 6.5).

FACILITATED STRETCHING

During facilitated stretching the muscle is lengthened to its comfortable limit and held for approximately 30 seconds. Then a static muscle

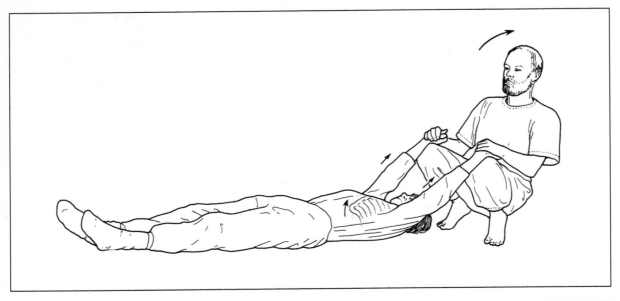

Fig. 6.5: Wrists on knees; improving respiration by opening rib cage with passive assisted stretching

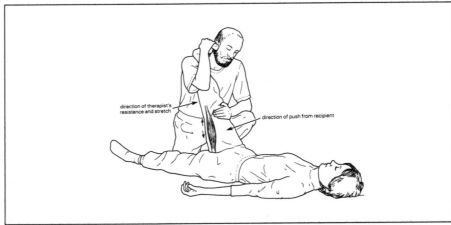

direction of therapist's resistance and stretch

direction of push from recipient

Fig. 6.6: Facilitated stretch on hamstrings

contraction is held for 6–10 seconds. The muscle is then relaxed and a passive assisted stretch is applied, during which the muscle will lengthen further.

The example in Fig. 6.6 shows a facilitated stretch applied to the Hamstring muscle group.

Each type of stretch has its relevant applications:

● All improve flexibility, especially facilitated stretching;
● All improve blood and lymphatic circulation, especially facilitated stretching because the contraction followed by lengthening has a pumping and flushing effect on the blood and lymph vessels, which also helps the breakdown and elimination of waste products accumulated within the muscle;
● A gravity stretch, or mild passive assisted stretch will bring a

Channel section which is kyo (and thus deeper) to the surface;

● For dispersing Jitsu areas, a facilitated stretch is required because the contraction phase will tire and therefore soften the muscle, allowing the muscle, and any Channel flowing through it to open more easily during the passive assisted phase, thus aiding the dispersal of blocked or overconcentrated Ki;

● All types of stretch can be applied to improve respiration, by opening the ribs.

Caution: Facilitated stretching should not be done extensively on Kyo Channels or with very weak and debilitated receivers. One or two gentle facilitated stretches are permissable on Kyo sections of a Channel in order to 'wake up' the area, provided they are followed by sustained perpendicular pressure to tonify.

Figs. 6.7 and 6.8 will give you various examples of stretching techniques:

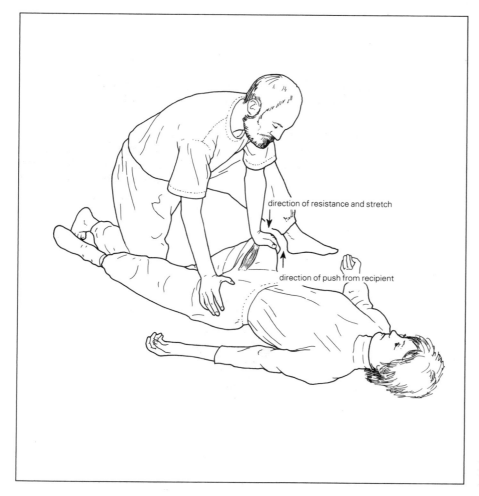

Improving Flexibility Using Facilitated Stretching

direction of resistance and stretch

direction of push from recipient

Fig. 6.7: Loosening hip adductors

**Improving Flexibility
Using Passive
Assisted Stretching**

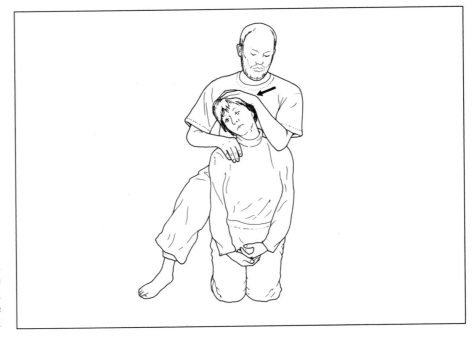

Fig. 6.8: Side Neck
stretch – this can be
done as a facilitated
stretch if extreme
caution is observed

IMPROVING BLOOD AND LYMPHATIC CIRCULATION – USING 'CROSS FIBRE' PASSIVE ASSISTED STRETCHING

All the flexibility techniques previously mentioned improve the circulation of blood and lymph. However, an especially effective method for decongesting the by-products of muscle metabolism, and therefore reducing the soreness and stiffness commonly experienced

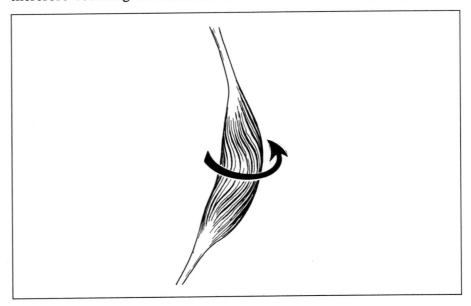

Fig. 6.9: Cross fibre
stretch to a muscle
belly

after strenuous exercise, is the 'cross fibre' passive assisted stretch. This technique is especially good for athletes and dancers.

A cross fibre stretch is a passive assisted stretch applied at right angles to the muscle fibres, a torsion which squeezes out stagnant waste products rather like wringing water out of a floor cloth (see Fig. 6.9).

Figs. 6.10 and 6.11 show a sequence of cross fibre stretching to relieve congestion in the thigh and calf.

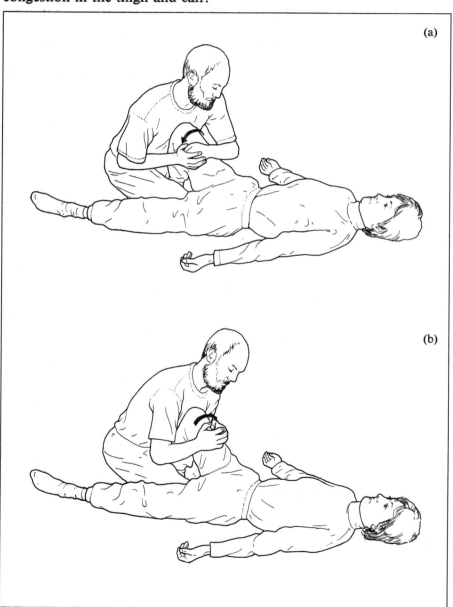

(a)

(b)

Fig. 6.10: Quadriceps

Fig. 6.11: Calf muscles

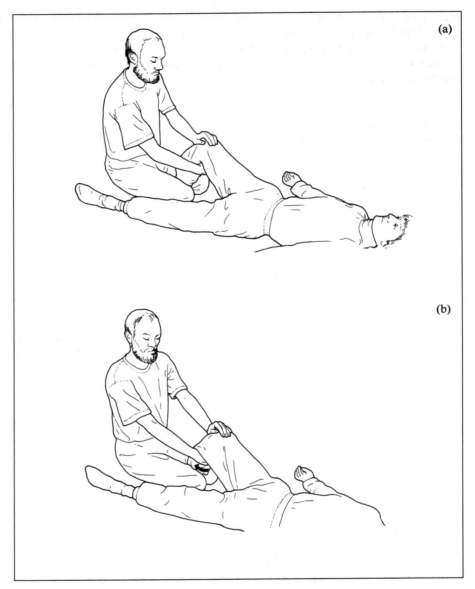

(a)

(b)

Cross fibre stretching applied to the general musculature on either side of the vertebral column is excellent for loosening stiff backs. This can be done by stretching the muscle away from the spine in prone lying, or in sitting (see Fig. 6.12).

Cross fibre can be done very locally with thumbs or fingertips, 'pushing and pulling' the muscle fibres rythmically. This is known as *Kenbiki* technique (see Fig. 6.13).

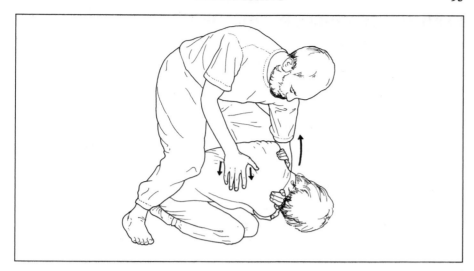

Fig. 6.12: Sitting with forward twist

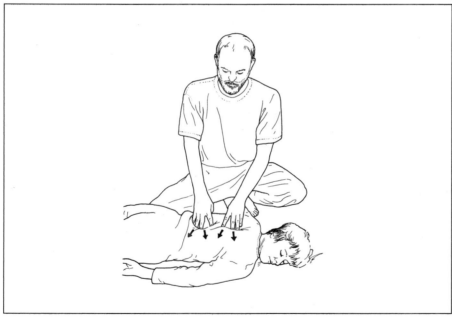

Fig. 6.13: Kenbiki applied to back muscles with fingertips. This technique can also be applied using the thumbs

BRINGING CHANNELS TO THE SURFACE

(Using gravity or passive assisted stretching)

Bringing a specific Channel to the surface within an arm or leg is simply achieved by placing the limb in a specific position. The required Channel can then be worked on more easily using less pressure. The stretch in itself 'opens' the Channel and encourages Ki to flow more smoothly. The following illustrations show these positions.

EXPOSING CHANNELS IN THE THIGH

Fig. 6.14: Channels in cross section viewed from above (left thigh)

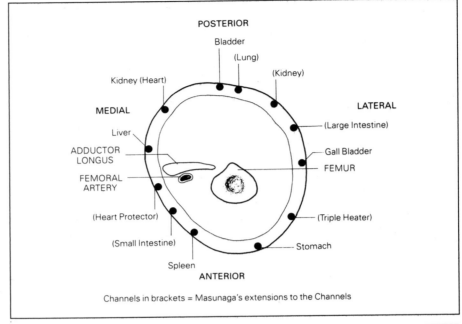

Channels in brackets = Masunaga's extensions to the Channels

Stretches in Supine

Fig. 6.15: Spleen

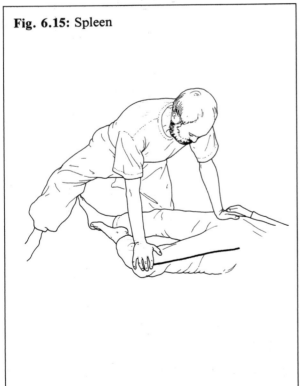

Fig. 6.16: Small Intestine extension

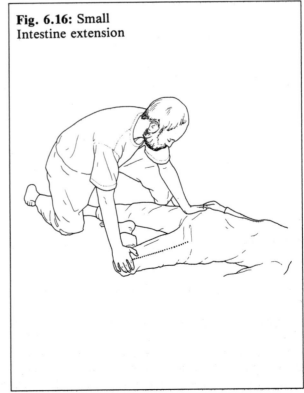

Fig. 6.17: Heart
Protector extension

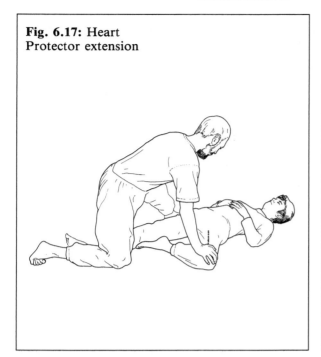

Fig. 6.18: Liver

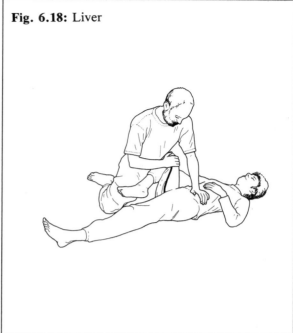

Fig. 6.19: Heart
extension

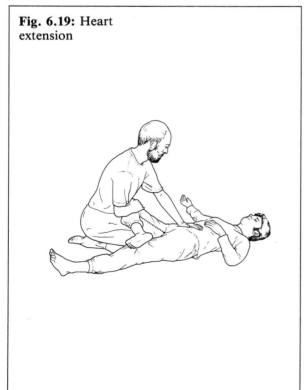

Fig. 6.20: Bladder

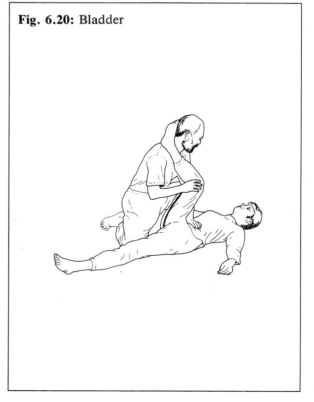

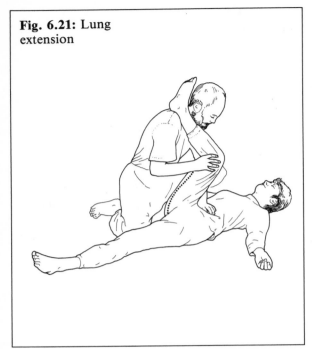

Fig. 6.21: Lung
extension

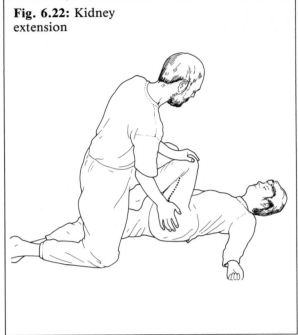

Fig. 6.22: Kidney
extension

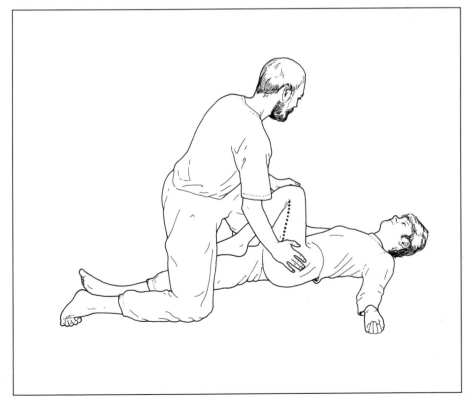

Fig. 6.23: Large
Intestine extension

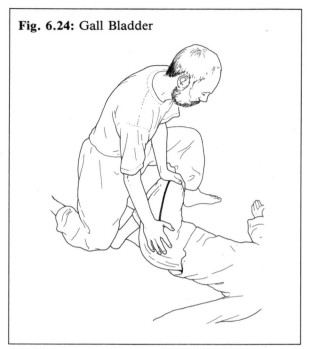

Fig. 6.24: Gall Bladder

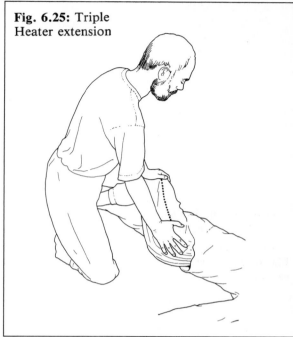

Fig. 6.25: Triple Heater extension

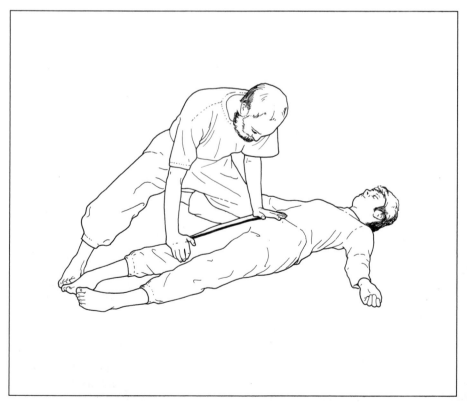

Fig. 6.26: Stomach (A)

Fig. 6.27: Stomach (B) Variation for more flexible recipients

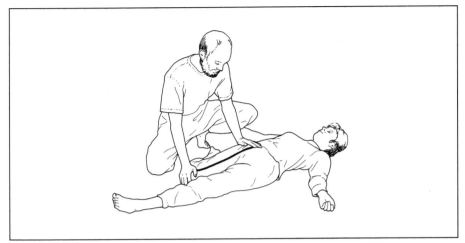

Stretches in Prone (below)

Fig. 6.28: Heart extension

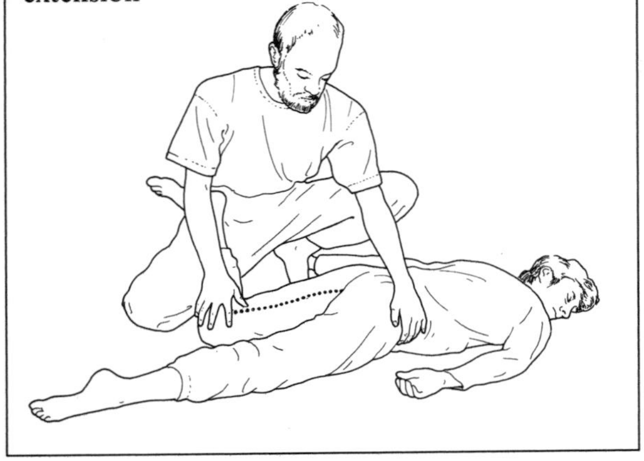

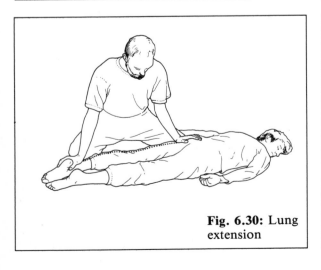

Fig. 6.29: Bladder

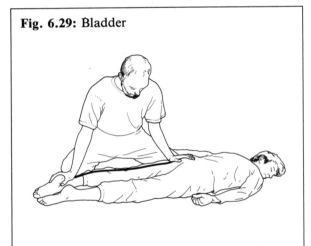

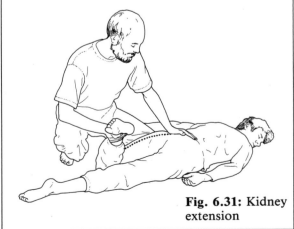

Fig. 6.30: Lung extension

Fig. 6.31: Kidney extension

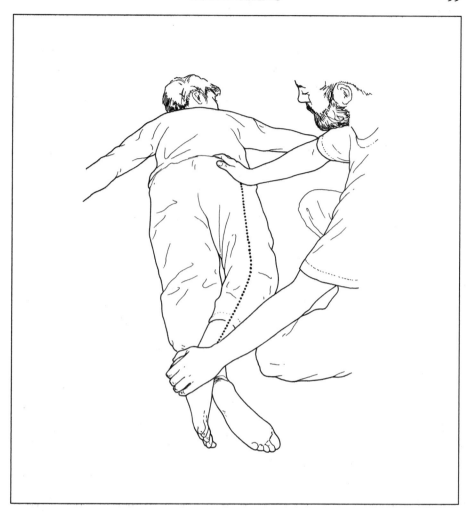

Fig. 6.32: Large
Intestine extension

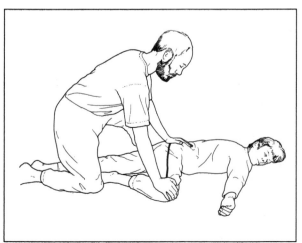

Fig. 6.33: Below left
Gall bladder

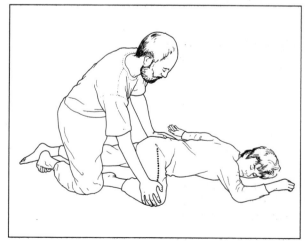

Fig. 6.34: Below Triple
Heater extension

Fig. 6.35: Stomach

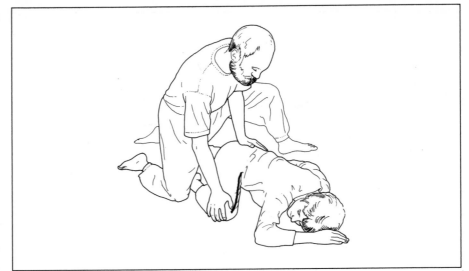

Stretches in Side Lying

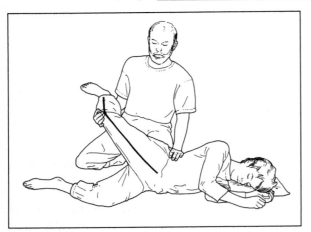

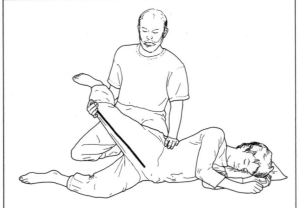

Fig. 6.36: Above
Stomach

Fig. 6.37: Above right
Spleen

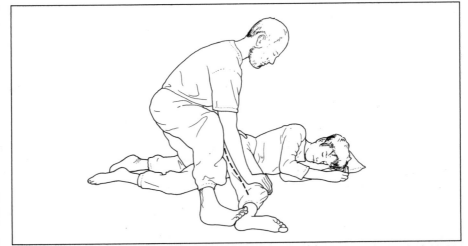

Fig. 6.38: Right
Bladder and Lung extension, and Kidney extension

Most of the lower leg Channels can be exposed with the same stretches as for the thigh. There is much less stretch occurring in the lower leg with these positions compared to the thigh, but the value lies in producing the optimum position to get at the Channels with correctly angled pressure.

EXPOSING CHANNELS IN THE ARM

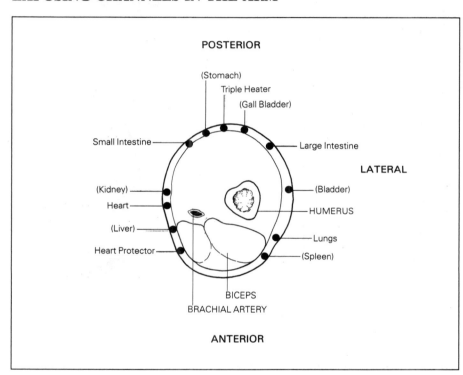

Fig. 6.39: Cross section from above, mid upper arm, left arm; lower arm is the same

Stretches in Supine

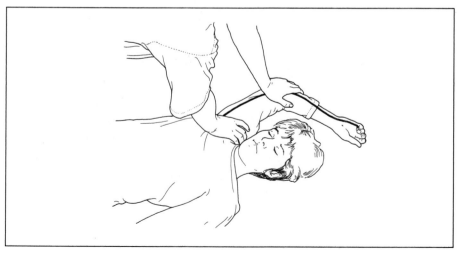

Fig. 6.40: Heart

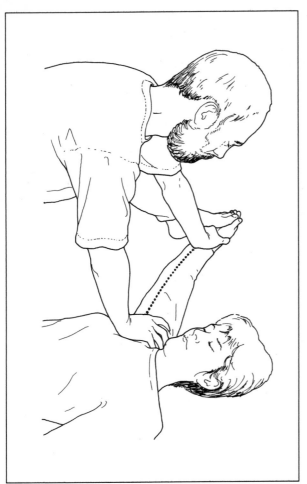

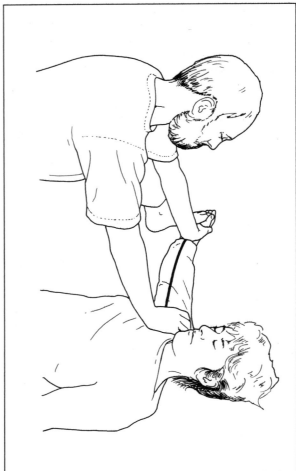

Fig. 6.41: Above Liver
extension

Fig. 6.42: Above right
Heart Protector

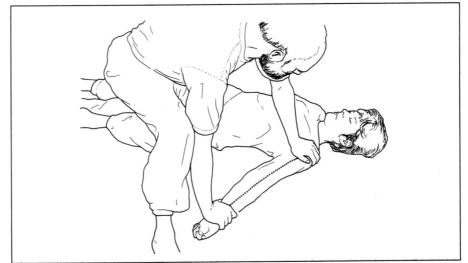

Fig. 6.43: Spleen
extension

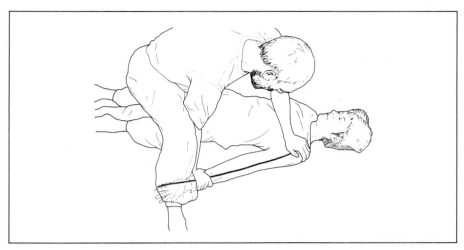

Fig. 6.44: Lung (N.B. Recipient's hand should be palm up)

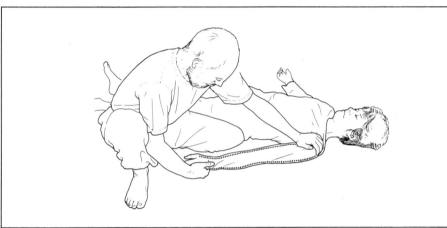

Fig. 6.45: Kidney/Bladder extensions (inner and outer edges of arms and forearms)

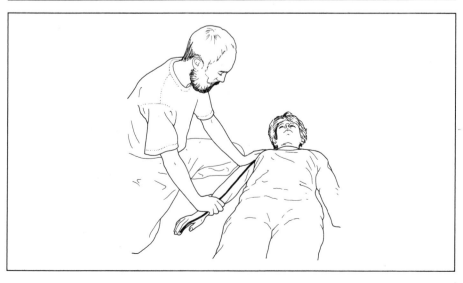

Fig. 6.46: Large Intestine

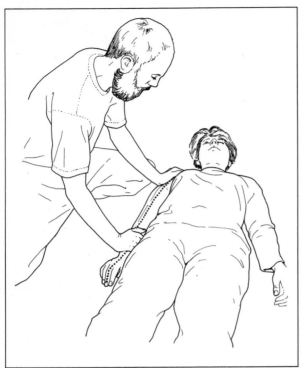

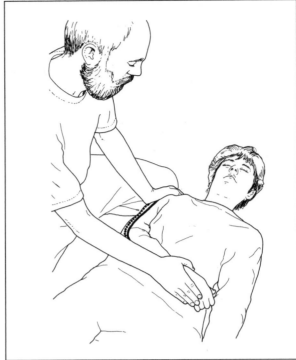

Fig. 6.47: Above Gall
Bladder extension

Fig 6.48: Above right
Triple Heater/Stomach
extension

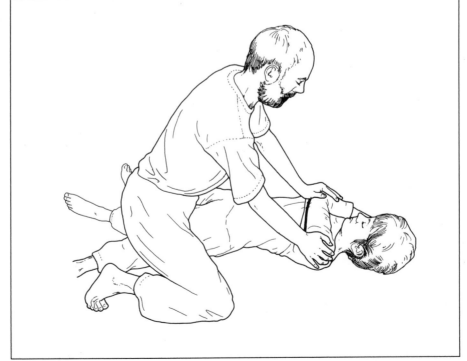

Fig. 6.49: Small
Intestine

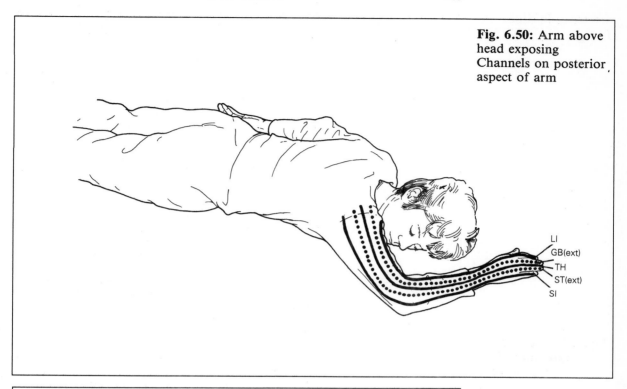

Fig. 6.50: Arm above head exposing Channels on posterior aspect of arm

LI
GB(ext)
TH
ST(ext)
SI

Stretches in Prone

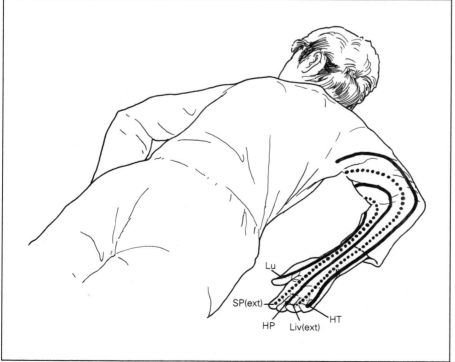

Lu
SP(ext)
HP   Liv(ext)   HT

Fig. 6.51: Arm by side exposing Channels on anterior aspect of arm

**Stretches in Side
Lying**

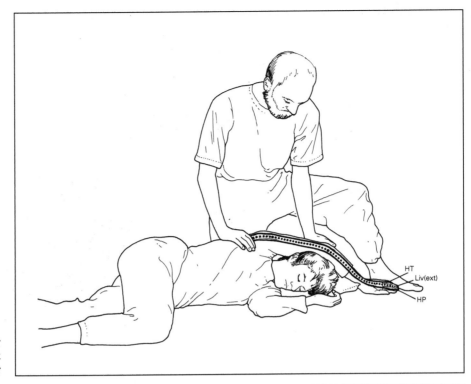

Fig. 6.52: Heart/Liver
extension/Heart
Protector

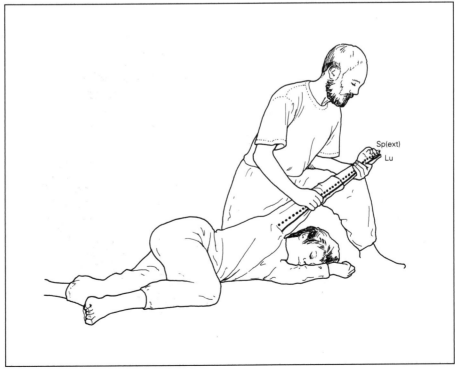

Fig. 6.53: Spleen
extension/Lung

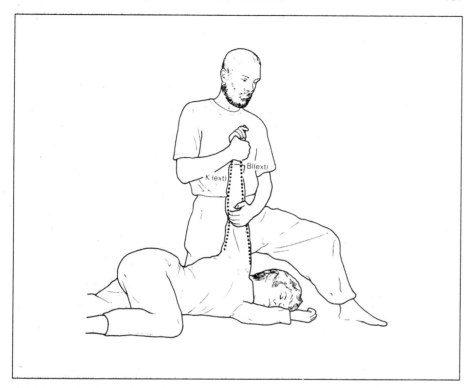

Fig. 6.54:
Kidney/Bladder
extensions

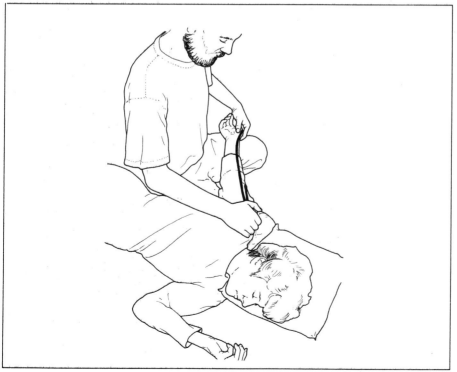

Fig. 6.55: Large intestine

Fig. 6.56: Gall Bladder
extension/Triple
Heater/Stomach
extension

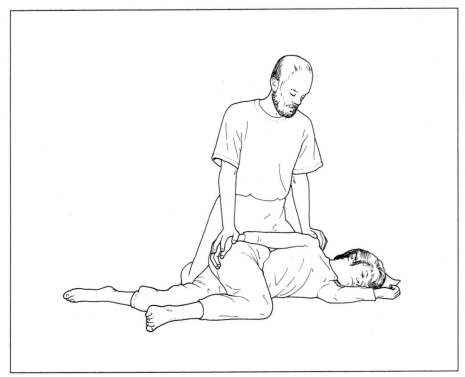

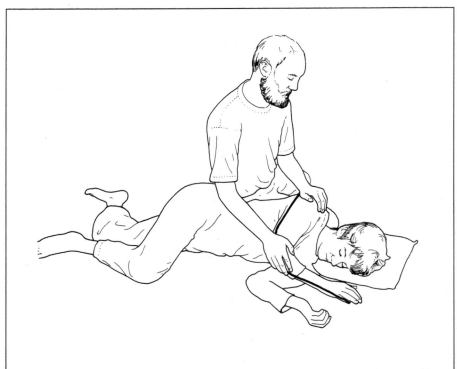

Fig. 6.57: Small
Intestine

With a little imagination, you can adapt the supine stretches for use in sitting (for example Fig 6.58). **Stretches in Sitting**

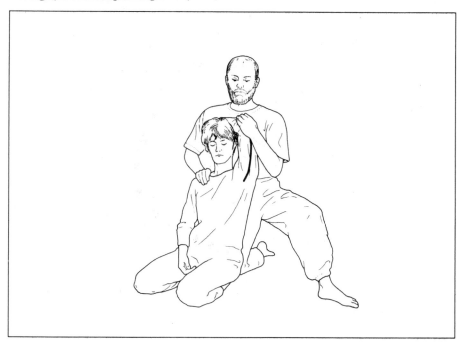

Fig. 6.58: Heart

EXPOSING CHANNELS IN TORSO

Generally, we simply have the receiver lying on his or her back to expose the Channels on the front of the torso, and have them lie on their front or side to expose the Channels on the back of the torso (see Fig. 6.59).

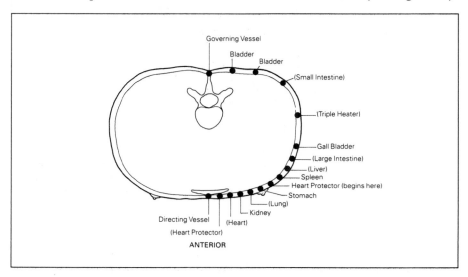

Fig. 6.59: Cross section through torso at nipple level, viewed from above

EXPOSING CHANNELS IN NECK

Fig. 6.60: Cross section through mid neck from above

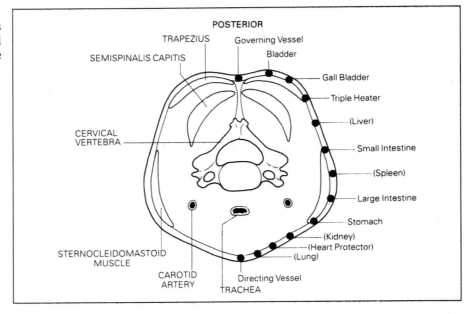

POSTERIOR

TRAPEZIUS — Governing Vessel
SEMISPINALIS CAPITIS — Bladder
— Gall Bladder
— Triple Heater
— (Liver)
CERVICAL VERTEBRA — Small Intestine
— (Spleen)
— Large Intestine
— Stomach
— (Kidney)
— (Heart Protector)
STERNOCLEIDOMASTOID MUSCLE — (Lung)
CAROTID ARTERY — Directing Vessel
TRACHEA

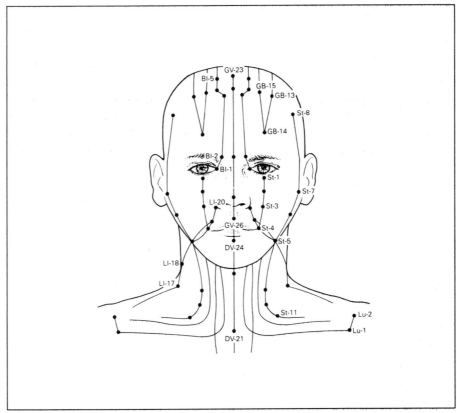

Bl-5 — GV-23
GB-15
GB-13
St-8
GB-14
Bl-2
Bl-1
St-1
LI-20
St-3
GV-26 — St-4
DV-24 — St-5
LI-18
LI-17
St-11
Lu-2
DV-21 — Lu-1

Fig. 6.61: Anterior aspect of neck

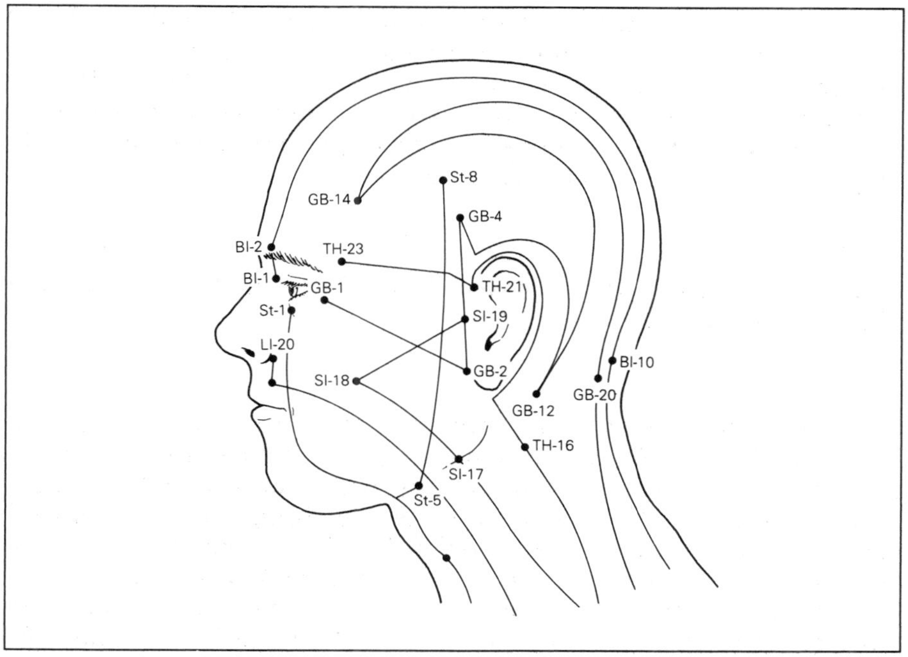

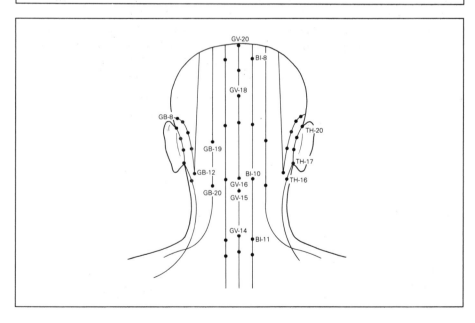

Fig. 6.62: Lateral aspect of neck

Fig. 6.63: Posterior aspect of neck

DISPERSING JITSU CHANNELS AND RELIEVING MUSCULAR TENSION USING FACILITATED STRETCHING

All the techniques described to improve flexibility and aid blood and lymphatic circulation can be used to disperse a Jitsu Channel section and relieve tense muscles. Similarly a facilitated stretch could be applied to many of the Channel opening positions. Bear in mind that tense muscles have an underlying cause which must be dealt with for maximum positive change. For example, tense shoulder and neck muscles may be due to emotional factors, or postural factors such as hip misalignment or a weak lumbar region.

OPENING THE RIB CAGE USING PASSIVE ASSISTED STRETCHING

Many people lack vitality simply because they fail to breathe to their full potential. This is partly the result of poor posture arising from a sedentary lifestyle, and partly due to being out of touch with their Hara – which is exacerbated by a sedentary lifestyle. Being out of touch with Hara immediately raises the centre of gravity so that the breathing becomes focused in the upper chest. It also makes one less able to maintain a state of relaxation in the face of routine stress factors, and more prone to emotional ups and downs. All these factors cause the breathing to be more shallow, quicker and more erratic.

It helps therefore, to assist the receiver to relax and become aware of their centre. Good general Shiatsu does this effectively. However, direct work on opening the rib cage can allow the receiver to experience what a deep breath is, maybe for the first time (see Figs 6.64 and 6.65).

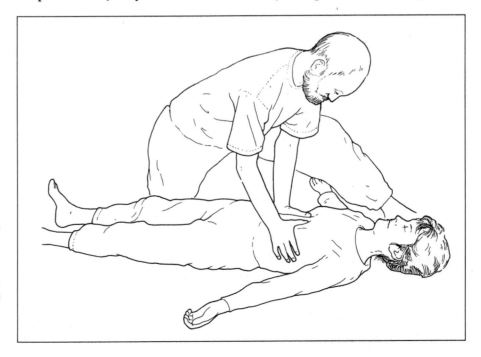

Fig. 6.64: Supine lying: lower rib press to extend exhalation, so that receiver automatically stretches ribs on resultant increased inhalation, thus encouraging awareness of breath in lower rib cage. Can be progressed by positioning arms over head

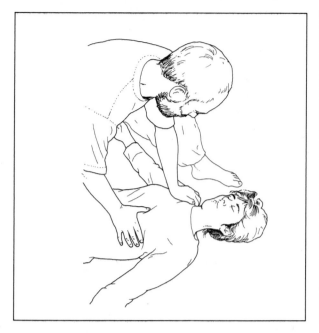 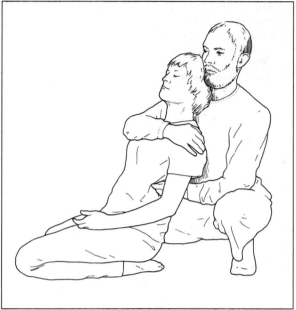

In the previous two examples a resistance could be applied during the inhalation phase. On release of pressure, the ribs will expand greatly and suddenly, bringing maximum air into the lungs.

Caution: This should be avoided in cases of high blood pressure, suspected weak ribs or asthma.

Fig. 6.65: Above left Supine lying: diagonal rib press; this and the previous technique can be done lying face down applying pressure to the back of the rib cage

Fig. 6.66: Above In sitting; 'Drape', using palms in back

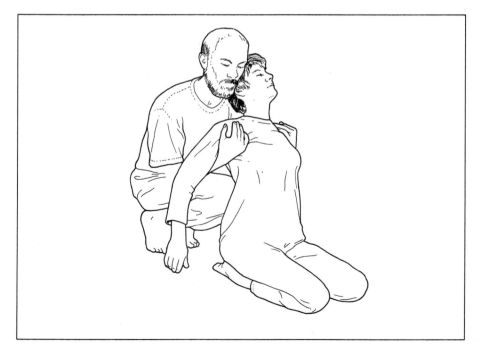

Fig. 6.67: Left In sitting; 'Drape', using knees in back (more powerful, can be painful)

Fig. 6.68: In sitting; receiver lies forward with arms supported by giver's thighs. Pressure applied to back with forearms

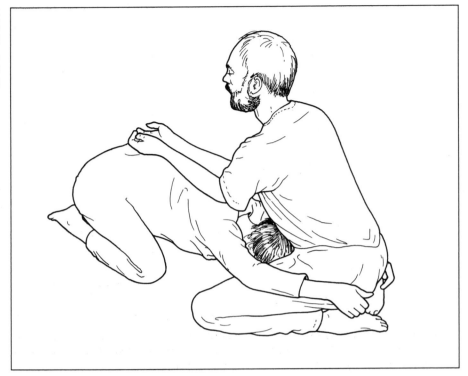

Fig. 6.69: In sitting; giver stands and stretches receiver's arms overhead, simultaneously easing thigh into back

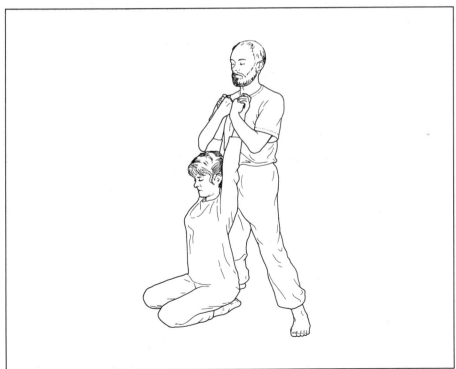

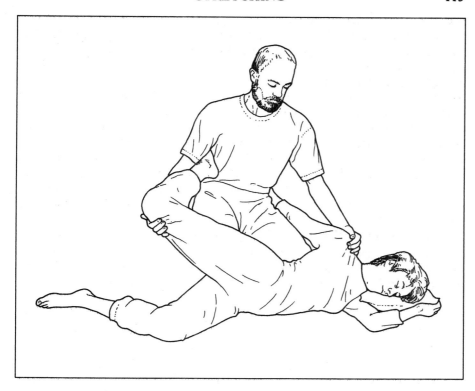

Fig. 6.70: In side lying; 'Bow' stretch (also an extreme stretch for the Stomach Channel)

A WORD ABOUT LIGAMENTS

A common misconception is that it is desirable to loosen the ligaments surrounding a joint to improve the range of movement a joint can

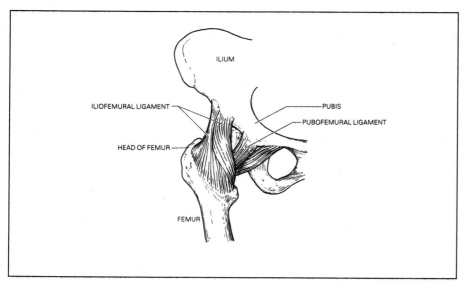

Fig. 6.71: Ligaments around the hip joint

perform. Nothing could be further from the truth. The range of movement any given joint is capable of is limited by tight muscles. The ligaments exist to support and stabilize the joint, thereby preventing excessive movement, or movement in undesirable directions. They literally strap the joint in place.

The ligaments have no elasticity and no ability to contract, being made of bands of connective tissue. If you stretch a ligament you will merely weaken it and make it more susceptible to tearing. Once stretched or torn, ligaments are extremely slow to repair because they have a very poor blood supply. Loose ligaments around a joint can render the joint liable to recurrent dislocation, as is common with the shoulder joint. Furthermore, the opposing joint surfaces can become mismatched, resulting in uneven wear and tear, and the consequent early onset of osteoarthritis.

A strong but flexible, elongatable musculature, with strong, firm ligaments is the ideal. Weak, loose muscles and loose ligaments are detrimental. However, there are circumstances when the joints are too tightly bound and congested, and require gentle mobilization.

PART 2

SHIATSU THERAPY AND ORIENTAL MEDICINE

Shiatsu is essentially a tactile, practical method for promoting health. One can practise Shiatsu with relatively little understanding of its theoretical basis. However, a solid grasp of its roots in Oriental Medicine will supplement intuitive skills and give an added depth of insight and confidence.

The application of the Kyo/Jitsu method in diagnosis and treatment can be very effective. However, this method in itself does not indicate the cause of an imbalance, nor the factors underlying the symptoms. Oriental Medicine provides a theoretical framework for understanding how physical and mental disharmonies originate and manifest.

The purpose of this section, therefore, is to present the fundamentals of Traditional Oriental Medicine. It includes those areas of Oriental Medicine important for a thorough knowledge of the causative patterns of disease and their alleviation through Shiatsu. Only such thorough knowledge will avoid the kind of misunderstanding and over-generalization to which Oriental Medicine is sometimes subject.

In practice, a Shiatsu therapist will tend to rely either more upon sensitivity and intuition, or upon reason and knowledge. The former type of practitioner will depend less upon their theoretical understanding and more upon their sensitivity to the flow of Ki. The latter type of practitioner will use a wider range of diagnostic skills and more frequently employ classical Tsubos. However, to rely exclusively on one approach or the other will limit the effectiveness of the treatment given. A well-rounded practitioner is one who realizes the full potential of Shiatsu through developing both sensitivity and theoretical insight. They are the practitioners who will ensure that Shiatsu therapy maintains a prominent position in natural medicine.

Chapter 7

Tao and Yin/Yang

TAO

Chinese Medicine evolved alongside the ancient philosophy of the *Tao*.
The Tao literally means a 'way' or a 'path'. To Taoists it came to mean
'The Way of the Universe'. One of its many observations is that all
phenomena are embraced by the Tao and so function ultimately as a
whole. All things in life can only be understood in relation to life in its
entirety.

Because the omnipresence of the Tao is a difficult concept to grasp, it
is seen as 'elusive and intangible',[1] 'dim and dark' to mind and
language. As the great sage Lao Tzu tells us in the Taoist classic, the *Tao
Te Ching*:

The Tao that can be told is not the eternal Tao.
The name that can be named is not the eternal name.[2]

The Tao is that 'irreducible dimension of the Real'[3] which cannot be
known or described through the analytical tool of words: it must be
apprehended through direct experience – it must be lived. It is at once
both hidden to one's mind and yet intimate with one's Being.

The Tao serves, sustains and yields to, rather than governs and
directs:

The ten thousand things depend on it: it holds nothing back.
It fulfils its purpose silently and makes no claim.[4]

Embracing all things and rejecting nothing, the Tao is a way of
expressing an Ultimate Reality which 'does not show greatness, and
therefore is truly great'. Instead of *exerting* power like the God of the
early Judaeo-Christian religions, it *contains* power like 'an empty vessel.
It is used, but never filled.'[5] Without effort, the Tao assumes the role of
a unifying principle only by virtue of its omnipresence:

Heaven's net casts wide.
Though its meshes are coarse, nothing slips through.[6]

Lao Tzu admonishes us to be 'at one with the Tao'. In Shiatsu, the
practitioner should allow him or herself to *yield* his or her energy to the

recipient in an effortless way; without straining or tensing, and without using overt physical force. Instead, gravity and body weight are used to apply pressure to the recipient, and the practitioner becomes, like the Tao, an 'empty vessel'.

From the perspective of the Tao, the practitioner will see the patient's disharmony as a part of the bodymind which has become detached from its true totality. The practitioner re-establishes harmony simply by helping the patient regain their innate oneness. 'The Tao of Heaven does not strive, and yet it overcomes.'

Disease in the Taoist vision is therefore seen as a situation where the individual is at some level 'out of step' with the dynamic, ever-changing, yet harmonious balance of Nature. This may be contrasted with Western scientific medicine which views disease as an invasive force unrelated and alien to the whole. In contrast, the Taoist believes that 'those who would conquer must yield'.[7]

The Tao is the source of all order; a cosmic order which is not static but organic in nature. It is complete in itself, and requires no doctrine in order to exist.

> You cannot improve it.
> If you try to change it, you will ruin it.
> If you try to hold it, you will lose it.[8]

The Tao guides without Laws or Commandments, and maintains harmony through 'Virtue', by which 'all things are nourished'. 'Virtue' is living according to the Tao:

> Creating without claiming,
> Doing without taking credit,
> Guiding without interfering.[9]

YIN/YANG

Yin/Yang are inseparable from the Tao: they are the two hands through which the Tao manifests and orders creation. Although they represent two polar antagonistic tendencies, they are complementary and interdependent. Everything in creation contains within it a Yin and Yang aspect; it is only in a relative sense that one thing is more Yin or Yang than another. The Yin/Yang dyad can be used to understand the relationship between any two structures, functions or processes. It forms the basis of Oriental Medicine.

The Yin aspect of a phenomenon is the structural and substantial; its Yang aspect is the active and energetic. Yin is therefore equated with the condensed and consolidated, dominated by the gravity of Earth. Yang mobilizes and expands, centrifugal in movement, associated with non-material existence or 'Heaven'.

Yin is like the ovum; Yang like the sperm. Yin remains a potential energy until it is activated by Yang. Thus, 'Heaven' acts on Earth, and Earth nourishes 'Heaven'. The two are interdependent; they flow into and contain each other, as illustrated in their symbol:

In terms of gender, Yin is considered to be more feminine, and Yang more masculine. However, just as it is incorrect to say a particular food is either Yin or Yang, it is equally misinformed to say that a woman is Yin and a man is Yang. All things are an interplay of both forces.

In the case of the human sexes, it is interesting to note that although women are outwardly more Yin, they contain within a more masculine unconscious which Carl Jung called the Animus. In turn, men possess a more feminine unconscious called the Anima. This is an example of the profound interdependence inherent in Yin/Yang.

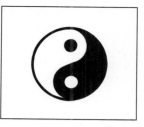

Fig. 7.1: Yin/Yang

YIN/YANG IN THE HUMAN BODY

In terms of bodily energetics, Chinese Medicine has selected four important Yin/Yang polarities and termed them the 'Eight Principles'. The Eight Principles provide the basic categories for the classification of bodily disharmonies.

The first two Principles provide a concept of bodily location in terms of Yin/Yang: these are Interior/Exterior. The Interior of the body is its more dense, Yin region, where the internal organs are located. The Exterior includes the relatively more superficial, Yang layers of the body; namely the skin and muscles. It is the more Yang role of the Exterior to protect the Interior. The Exterior protects the body from pathogenic factors such as Cold and Dampness which tend to invade the body from the outside. Diseases which are due to pathogenic invasion are called 'Exterior conditions'. These types of conditions always require Shiatsu treatment which is dispersing in style, in order to help the body drive out the unwanted pathogens.

Interior/Exterior

Problems which arise from within, whether chronic or acute, are in turn called 'Interior conditions'. They may require either tonification or dispersal, depending on the particular condition involved.

Although not included among the 'Eight Principles', another polarity of body location is superior/inferior. Because Yang describes upward-moving energy and Yin downward, the upper parts of the body are more Yang and the lower more Yin. The brain, at the more Yang superior pole of the body, is concerned with more rarefied, subtle and Yang phenomena; namely nervous stimuli and thought. The intestines, in a relatively more Yin inferior position, accordingly deal with more coarse, dense and Yin phenomena.

Hot/Cold The second Eight Principle polarity is Hot/Cold. Normal body function requires internal warmth not only for comfort, but for its many different transformative functions. Processes of warming and transformation (e.g. of food into Blood) belong to the Yang function of the body. They find their source in the 'Gate of Vitality' ('Ming Men') provided by the Yang (energetic) aspect of the Kidneys and located near the Tsubo Governor Vessel-4.

In contrast, it is the role of the Yin of the body to cool, calm and moisten. The body's Yin is derived from the Yin aspect of the Kidneys and from the Stomach, which, because of its role in digestion, is the source of the Body Fluids.

When, for a variety of possible reasons, the body's warming functions are over-stimulated, often at the expense of its cooling ones, a Hot condition arises. The signs of internal Heat include thirst, possible fever, restlessness, a rapid pulse, a red face and tongue, and scanty, dark urine. They indicate a relative excess of Yang in the body. If on the other hand, the body's warming functions become impaired, a Cold condition arises, involving signs which include chilliness, a lack of thirst, a pale face and tongue, and abundant, clear urine. They indicate a relative excess of Yin.

Full/Empty The Eight Principle categories of Full/Empty provide another important way of assessing the condition of the body. A Full or 'Excess' condition is one which is characterized by an excess of such things as Yin or Yang (see fig. 7.2 opposite), Ki, Blood or Body Fluids, as described in chapter 8, or external causes of disease such as Heat, Cold, Wind, Damp, Fire, all of which are described fully in chapter 9. The general signs of a full condition include a sudden, acute onset of symptoms with pain made worse by pressure, profuse sweating, irritability, and a strong voice.

An Empty or 'Deficient' condition is characterized by a depletion of Yin or Yang (see fig. 7.2 opposite) or of Ki, Essence, Blood or Body Fluids (see chapter 8); either generally or within a particular organ, e.g. Spleen Ki Deficiency (see page 168), Kidney Essence Deficiency (see page 148). The general signs of an Empty condition can include chronic disease with pain alleviated by pressure, slight sweating, listlessness, and a weak voice. In reality, most disharmonies include signs of both a Full and Empty character, although one of the two usually predominate.

Emptiness of Ki and/or Blood commonly leads to areas of the body such as the Hara exhibiting a loss of muscular tone, and showing a lack of resistance to pressure. Emptiness of Yang in the body will add paleness and coldness to these signs.

The last two Eight Principle categories are Yin and Yang themselves, and generally serve to summarize the ones we have already discussed.

There are three Yin/Yang diagnostic classifications which are found in practice: these are (1) Empty Yang; (2) Excess Yang; and (3) Empty Yin. Excess Yin is not generally considered to be a common occurrence, as it results only from exposure to extremes of cold.

When Yang becomes excessive, the body generates heat and becomes hyperactive. This is Excess Yang. Alternatively, a Hot condition may also arise because of a lack of cool, moist Yin energy in the body, allowing the Yang to predominate and so generate heat and dryness. This is Empty Yin. The following graphs illustrate and compare Empty Yang with Excess Yang, as well as the important distinction between Excess Yang and Empty Yin.

Yin/Yang Balance

Fig. 7.2: A graph of Yin/Yang combinations

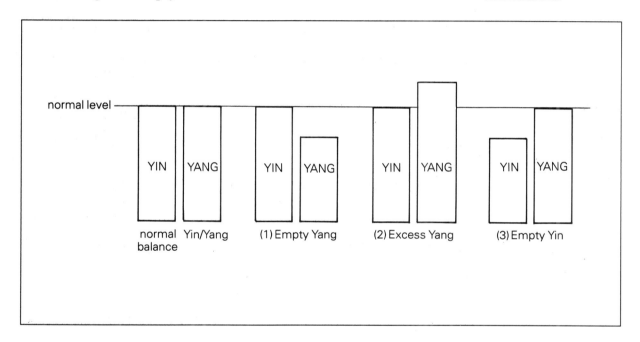

Let us now summarize these three basic states of bodily disharmony by comparing their signs and symptoms.

Empty Yang	Excess Yang	Empty Yin
tired	restless	restless but underlying weakness
sleeps heavily	can't get to sleep/restless sleep	gets to sleep but wakes frequently
cold	hot	hot hands and feet
cold day and night	hot day and night	hot mainly during afternoon/night
no thirst	strong thirst	thirst mainly during afternoon/night
pale face	red face	red cheeks ('malar flush')
pale tongue with white coating	red tongue with yellow coating	bright red thin tongue (no coating)
copious, clear urine	scanty, dark urine	scanty, dark urine
loose stools	constipated with possible pain	dry stools with no pain
listless	agitated	anxious
unconfident	arrogant	defensive
apathetic	driven	over-extended

Finally, Yin/Yang is used to classify the internal organs into pairs, each pair sharing the same Element. The Yin (or 'Zang') organs are those which are relatively more solid in structure. They 'store the precious Substances' (i.e. the Essence, Ki, Blood and pure Body Fluids). The Yang (or 'Fu' organs) are considered 'hollow workshop organs', and are responsible for the transportation and excretion of bodily substances. Each pair of organs are interdependent. Although the most important body functions belong to the Yin organs, the Channels of both the Yin and Yang organs are of equal importance in Shiatsu therapy.

Element	Yin (Zang) Organ	Yang (Fu) Organ
Water	Kidneys	Bladder
Wood	Liver	Gall Bladder
Fire	Heart	Small Intestines
	Heart Governor	Triple heater
Earth	Spleen	Stomach
Metal	Lungs	Large Intestines

NOTES

1. *Tao Te Ching* by Lao Tzu, translated by Gia-Fu Feng and Jane English, Vintage Books, 1972, ch. 21.
2. *Tao Te Ching*, ch. 1.
3. *Survey of Traditional Chinese Medicine*, by Claude Larre, Jean Schatz and Elisabeth Rochat de la Vallee, translated by Sarah Elizabeth Stang, Institut Ricci, Paris, and Traditional Acupuncture Institute, U.S.A., 1986, p.39.
4. *Tao Te Ching*, ch. 24.
5. *Tao Te Ching*, ch. 4.
6. *Tao Te Ching*, ch. 73.
7. *Tao Te Ching*, ch. 61.
8. *Tao Te Ching*, ch. 29.
9. *Tao Te Ching*, ch. 51.

Chapter 8

The Vital Substances

At the basis of Oriental Medicine are the four fundamental Substances of the bodymind: Ki, Blood, 'Essence' (Jing) and Body Fluids. The word 'substance' is possibly misleading, as they should really be viewed as vital forces, each varying in the amount of actual 'substance' it possesses. Of the four, Ki is the most rarefied and active; hardly a 'substance' at all. Blood is relatively more material in form, yet helps the Heart to house the Mind. The Essence is the most concentrated of the vital substances – a type of 'essential energy'.[1] The Body Fluids are also material in form, yet even they possess energetic importance.

'Mind' (Shen) may be considered a type of Ki – the most refined of all. 'Shen' has often been translated as 'Spirit', but the Shen does not in fact refer to the primarily 'spiritual' aspect of an individual. Shen is something much more fundamental: it is one's day-to-day consciousness and all that this entails. It embraces thoughts, feelings, dreams and perceptions of every possible kind; not just those of a 'spiritual' nature. The Mind will be discussed in detail in Chapter 13.

The concept of Ki   Ki (Qi in Chinese) is generally translated as 'energy'. However, a look at the Chinese character for Ki reveals that it has two different aspects: a component which represents a 'vapour' or 'gas' and one that means 'rice'. These symbols express its material and immaterial manifestations. Also, the vapour represents the air we breathe and the rice, the food we eat; together they form bodily Ki.

Ki forms the very basis of all phenomena in the universe and affords a continuum between crude substance and subtle, invisible force. It animates and moves, changing constantly, gathering and dispersing in life's perpetual play.

The concept of bodily Ki is relatively more specific but no less fundamental. According to the *Nan Jing* (AD 100), 'Ki is the root of a human being.' It governs all the body's processes, both physical and mental, and thus appears as different types of Ki varying in location and function.

ESSENCE

'Essence' or 'Jing' is Ki at its most dense. It is formed at conception and nourishes the foetus during pregnancy, depending on the mother's Kidneys for sustenance. One might think of it as genetic in origin. This so-called 'Pre-Heaven Essence' accounts for individual constitutional strength and resistance to disease. Because it is inherited from one's parents, it is generally fixed in quantity and quality. However, overwork, poor diet and excessive sexual activity over a long period will contribute to the early depletion of Pre-Heaven Essence. On the other hand, it can be strengthened through special ways of cultivating Ki such as Tai Ji Quan, Qi Gong and Yoga.

The term 'Post-Heaven Essence' is given to the Essence which is extracted from food and refined by the Stomach and Spleen after birth. It replenishes the Pre-Heaven Essence stored in the Kidneys, and together they produce the generalized Essence which, due to its fluid nature, is able to circulate throughout the body.

The Essence has a number of functions all concerned with growth, reproduction and development, as well as sexual maturation, conception and pregnancy. It is said to fill 'The Sea of Bone Marrow', consisting not only of the bones but of the brain, spinal cord and teeth as well.

The Essence therefore determines proper growth and development of the entire individual, particularly of the bones, teeth and hair. It also provides the basis for normal brain development. According to the *Nei Ching*, the Essence of a man follows an eight-year cycle, while the Essence of a woman follows a seven-year cycle. In this way, the Essence controls the development of sexual characteristics, reproductive function and fertility. Without the Essence, conception and pregnancy would be impossible. Finally, it determines the natural decline of sexual energy and fertility in the ageing process.

As the Essence is stored in the Kidneys, it interacts closely with the Yin, Yang and Ki of the Kidneys.

Picture the Kidneys as a cauldron full of water: The fire under the cauldron is produced by the Kidney-Yang and the 'Gate of Vitality' ('Ming Men') located at the Tsubo Governor Vessel-4; the water contained by the cauldron may be thought of as the Kidney-Essence and Kidney-Yin; and the steam produced by the heating of the water represents the Kidney-Ki which results from the process. Kidney-Ki thus ascends to the Lungs, which are responsible for its dispersal around the body (see Fig. 8.1).

In short, the Essence provides the Kidney-Yin with the necessary substance to form Kidney-Ki through the warming action of Kidney-Yang.

Finally, due to its 'genetic' nature, the Essence accounts for our underlying constitutional strength and resistance to disease. If the Essence is deficient at birth, or becomes depleted later in life, a number of possible problems may manifest. Those problems related to growth,

Fig. 8.1: Kidney 'cauldron'

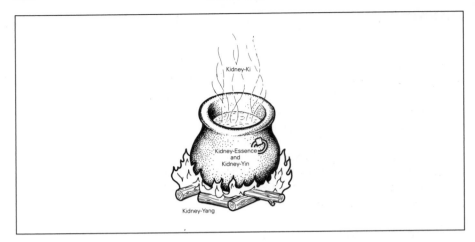

reproduction and development include retarded growth in children, malformation of bones, infertility, repeated miscarriage, loose teeth, loss of hair and premature ageing. Those problems directly involving the Kidneys include lower back pain, poor sexual vitality and hearing problems. If a deficiency of Essence affects the 'Sea of Bone Marrow' (which includes the brain), there may be a lack of concentration and memory as well as dizziness and tinnitus (ringing in the ears). In a general sense, the Essence contributes to the vitality of Ki and clarity of the mind; a deficiency will mean susceptibility to disease and mental fatigue.

The strength of the Essence may be assessed from the patient's medical history. A further sign of poor constitution is the absence of complete and detached earlobes: if the lobes are attached to the skin or virtually absent, it may be taken as another indication that the Essence should be cultivated.

KI

There are a number of types of Ki, all with different bodily and energetic functions. Its functions include the transformation of food into energy and Blood, the transportation of Fluids, holding the Organs in place, and the protecting and warming of the body.

The following explanation of the various types of Ki illustrates the detail with which Oriental Medicine explains the transformation of Ki within the body.

The first type of Ki is Original Ki. Original Ki stems directly from the Essence; in fact, it is Essence in the form of Ki, and can be considered our constitutional energy. Original Ki is the motivating force behind every function in the body. It acts as a catalyst for the creation of all the other types of Ki, as well as for the transformation of Food into Blood. It thus forms the basis of bodily vitality and endurance.

Original Ki is the foundation of the Hara and resides at its very centre, in the Gate of Vitality. The Gate of Vitality lies below the navel, between the Kidneys, and is the source-point of the body's energy and warmth. It is associated with two main Tsubos: Directing Vessel-6 (the lower 'Sea of Ki') and Governing Vessel-4 ('Ming Men' or 'Gate of Vitality'). Tonification of these points will directly reinforce the Gate of Vitality and the Original Ki. Like the Essence, the Original Ki is closely connected to the Kidneys, and provides the basis of Kidney-Ki. However, it is the job of the Triple Heater to spread the Original Ki from the Gate of Vitality to the internal Organs and their twelve main channels, where it surfaces at the Source Points.

Food Ki is produced by the Stomach and Spleen through the transformation of food into energy. However, Food Ki cannot be utilized by the body until it rises to the chest and combines with air to form Gathering Ki. It is the Spleen's function to raise the Food Ki to the chest where, with the help of the Original Ki, Food Ki is transformed into Blood.

Gathering Ki, also called Chest Ki, is a combination of Food Ki and Air Ki. It is a more refined and rarefied form of Ki than Food Ki and is therefore more easily utilized by the body. It vitalizes the Lungs and Heart, gives strength to the voice and invigorates the circulation of blood. It is located at the Tsubo Directing Vessel-17 (the upper 'Sea of Ki') and may be tonified through stimulation of this point.

Gathering Ki gives rise to True Ki under the motivating power of Original Ki. True Ki is the last stage in the transformation of Ki from its relatively crude state as Original Ki. Like Gathering Ki, True Ki is governed by the Lungs, the main function of which is to control Ki as a whole. True Ki manifests in two different forms; Nutritive Ki and Defensive Ki.

Nutritive Ki circulates in the Channels and blood vessels and, together

Fig. 8.2:
Transformation of Ki

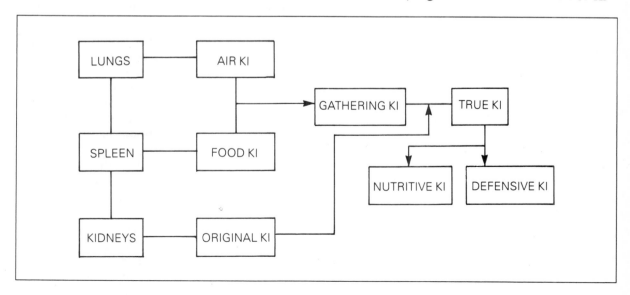

with the blood, supplies the body with nourishment. Defensive Ki is more Yang in relation to Nutritive Ki and circulates around the periphery of the body in the space between the muscles and skin. It acts as a protective barrier to the external world. Whereas Nutritive Ki is located in the interior and nourishes the body, Defensive Ki flows on the Exterior and protects it.

Whenever the body is exposed to external pathogenic factors such as Heat, Cold, Wind and Damp, the Defensive Ki acts like a shield to block their invasive power. It has the further function of warming and moistening the skin and muscles, opening and closing the pores, and therefore of regulating body temperature.

Both the skin and the muscles are controlled by the Lungs. It is therefore not surprising that a weakness of Lung Ki can lead to a weakness of Defensive Ki, and make one more susceptible to colds and flu. However, it should be noted that the Defensive Ki is also supported by the Kidney-Ki and is nourished by the Spleen and Stomach.

BLOOD

The Blood has wider connotations in Oriental Medicine than in Western understanding. Apart from transporting the body's nourishment, the Blood also plays a role in housing the Mind.

The process of Blood formation begins with the Spleen, which transforms and refines food and liquid into Food Ki, the basis of Blood. From the Spleen Food Ki is raised by the Lungs to the Heart. Here, with the help of the Original Ki, it is transformed into Blood. Although the Spleen is the origin of Blood, it is the Heart which 'governs' the Blood, mainly because it is responsible for its circulation. However, the Spleen also plays an important role in keeping the Blood in the blood vessels; it 'controls' the Blood.

Apart from providing the Original Ki necessary for Blood formation, the Kidneys play a further role through their production of the Bone Marrow, which also contributes to the manufacture of Blood.

The Liver is not directly involved in the production of Blood but is responsible for the storage of Blood during times of sleep and rest. When the body is in a horizontal position, a large proportion of the Blood goes to the Liver to be stored, and only circulates again when the body is active.

Finally, it should be noted that the Blood has a close interdependent relationship with the Ki. Not only is Ki crucial to Blood formation, but is also necessary for the circulation of Blood through the vessels: the Ki moves the Blood.

BODY FLUIDS

Body Fluids are the product of food and drink which have been transformed and separated by the Spleen and Stomach. The 'clean' fluids are transported to the Lungs. The Lungs then disperse them around the body and under the skin, as well as down to the Kidneys.

The 'dirty' portion of the fluids we take are further refined by the Small Intestines; the pure portion goes to the Bladder for its excretion as perspiration and urine, and the impure portion is excreted by the Large Intestines. Some water is reabsorbed by the Large Intestines and goes to the Bladder, mainly for excretion.

The Spleen is the most important organ in relation to the Body Fluids, as it ensures that the pure fluids move upwards for dissemination by the Lungs, and the impure fluids move downwards for excretion by the Bladder. When a Ki- or Yang-deficient Spleen fails to transform fluids as it should, an excessive build-up of Body Fluids will lead to Damp or Phlegm accumulation. It is usually necessary to treat the Spleen in this instance.

The Kidneys also play a vital role in the control of Body Fluids. First, they help to remove impure fluids from the body. Secondly, they vaporize some of the fluids they receive and send them up to the Lungs, helping to keep the Lungs moist. Finally, they supply the Bladder, their paired Organ, with the necessary Ki to transform fluids into sweat and urine.

The Lungs 'dominate the Water passages' through their function of dispersing and descending – dispersing Body Fluids throughout the body to the space beneath the skin, and descending them to the Kidneys. (Note that the Kidneys and Lungs have a reciprocal relationship: the Kidneys vaporize the Body Fluids and send them up to the Lungs for dispersal; the Lungs send down Body Fluids to the Kidneys for their excretion.)

Finally, the Organ of Triple Heater plays an important supportive role in the physiology of Body Fluids. It is said in *The Yellow Emperor's Classic* that 'The Triple Heater is the official in charge of irrigation, and controls the water passages.' The Upper Heater, likened to a 'mist', helps the Lungs in its dispersing and descending functions, as well as the Spleen in its job of 'raising the Food-Ki'. The Middle Heater, compared to a 'muddy pool', assists the Stomach in churning the fluids and sending the 'dirty' portion downwards. The Lower Heater is like a 'drainage ditch' because it helps the Kidneys, Bladder and Small Intestines separate and excrete fluids. It is the Triple Heater which orchestrates these many processes, and ensures the availability of the Original Ki necessary to effect them.

Thus, the Body Fluids are like the Blood: both are closely dependent upon the Ki for their transformation and transportation. In turn, they support the Ki through nourishing and moistening the Organs which produce, disseminate and regulate Ki.

Chapter 9

The Causes of Disease

The causes of disease in Oriental Medicine are categorized according to those which are Internal (i.e. emotional); those which are External (i.e. climatic); and those which are miscellaneous.

THE INTERNAL CAUSES OF DISEASE

In Oriental Medicine there is a direct relationship between the emotional life of a person and their physical health. Each internal Organ is closely associated with a range of associated emotions. The Organs dominate the expression of particular emotions and their function is in turn affected by them. For example, a disharmony of the Lungs will lead to sadness and melancholy; conversely, always feeling sad will weaken the Lungs. Thus, in diagnosis, little distinction is ultimately made between the mind and the body. Remembering this, it is easy to understand how certain emotions can play a role in the causation of disease.

The seven basic emotions which make up the Internal Causes of Disease are:

- Fear
- Anger
- Joy
- Shock or Fright
- Worry
- Pensiveness
- Sadness

These terms are broad categories and include a wide range of associated feelings. In normal circumstances they play a generally positive role in the life of bodymind. They only exert a negative influence when they become too intense or dominate the psyche over a long period of time.

Fear   An appropriate sense of instinctive fear is important for survival. However, excessive or prolonged fear makes the Ki descend and drains the Kidneys. In particular, fear depletes the Kidneys of Yin, causing Heat in the Heart and related emotions such as anxiety and insecurity.

Anger

Anger is sometimes necessary to exert one's authority. However, excessive and inappropriate anger make the Ki rise and causes Stagnation or Heat in the Liver. Headaches, indigestion and other problems commonly result. The term Anger here may include a number of associated feelings such as frustration, irritability and resentment.

Joy

Joy in general is naturally beneficial to one's emotional well-being. What can be damaging is over-excitement and an abnormal degree of mental stimulation, both of which are forms of excessive 'Joy'. This type of excessive Joy slows down the Ki.

Shock

Mental shock scatters the Ki and adversely affects both the Kidneys and Heart. The Ki of the Heart is rapidly weakened and requires the Kidney-Essence to support it. This in turn puts a strain on the Kidneys.

Worry and Pensiveness

Worry and pensiveness (excessive thinking) are said to 'knot' the Ki, thereby disrupting the flow of Ki in the spleen and, to some extent, the Lungs. Because the Spleen houses Thought, it is particularly affected by thinking which is obsessive and fraught with over-concern. The Spleen's central role in digestion becomes disrupted and Dampness accumulates in the body. The Lungs react to worry by causing difficulty in breathing.

Sadness

The Lungs when in a state of harmony are the source of vitality and optimism. However, when we are overcome with sadness and grief the Lungs are weakened. Because the Lungs govern the Ki, sadness 'dissolves' Ki and tiredness results. Moreover, it is now well known that prolonged depression weakens the immune system. This can be explained by the fact that the Lungs also govern the Defensive Ki.

THE EXTERNAL CAUSES OF DISEASE

Whereas the Internal Causes of Disease are relatively subtle and arise from within, the External Causes are of a physical nature and encroach upon the body from the environment. They are referred to as 'external pathogenic factors' and are climatic in origin. They include:

- Wind
- Cold
- Heat/Fire
- Summer-Heat
- Dryness
- Dampness

Susceptibility to these pathogenic factors depends both on the strength of their impact on the body, and the body's strength in resisting them. Living in a region of extreme weather conditions will make diseases of an External origin common. However, those with a poor constitution and weak Defensive Ki will fall prey to the same diseases in a similar but less extreme climatic region.

These climatic terms refer both to the origin of the symptoms and the type of symptoms that are manifesting. They are primarily used as a means of classifying disharmonies which are caused by the physical environment. All disharmonies of an External origin are Excess conditions. There may be an underlying deficiency of Ki which allows external pathogenic factors to penetrate, but they are Excess in nature because they must be dispelled before the body can recover.

Wind   Whereas the other External causes of disease are more closely related to specific climatic influences, the term 'Wind' indicates a pattern of disharmony rather than a climatic factor. Wind is characterized by symptoms which in modern terms would be labelled as a cold or flu. At the onset of these symptoms, 'Wind' invades the body and penetrates to the Exterior level between the skin and muscles, where the Defensive Ki circulates. Because the Lungs are the most 'external' Organ of the body, and because they control the Defensive Ki, they are the first Organ to be affected by an invasion of Wind. Wind affects the dispersing and descending function of the Lungs, causing sneezing, blocked sinuses, muscular aching, headaches and an aversion to cold.

Wind is characterized by acute symptoms which reflect the action of wind in nature: it arises swiftly, changes quickly, and blows forcefully and sporadically. Climatic wind makes the trees shake and sway; pathogenic Wind causes shivering. Wind is Yang in nature and therefore tends to injure the Yin.

The presence of External Wind is indicated by a Floating pulse (see p.212), as the Ki rises to the superficial Defensive level of the body in order to fight off the pathogenic factor. There are two types of external wind: Wind-Cold and Wind-Heat.

Wind-Cold   Wind-Cold is characterized by sneezing, shivering, an aversion to cold, cough, and a runny nose with white or clear mucous. There is also likely to be stiffness and aching (especially in the neck and back of the head), a light fever, and an absence of sweating or thirst. An invasion of Wind-Cold results in a pulse which is both Floating and Tight.

Wind-Heat is characterized by feverishness and sweating, thirst, cough, **Wind-Heat** and nasal congestion with yellow mucus. A sore throat and headache are also likely to arise. In comparison to Wind-Cold, muscular aching and aversion to cold will be mild, whereas fever will be heavy. Wind-Heat results in a pulse which is both Floating and Rapid.

External Cold may penetrate into the body of those people who live or **Cold** work in cold conditions. It is also more likely among people who do not, or cannot, dress properly. Cold causes Ki-stagnation and results in contraction of the muscles and joints, cramping pain and watery discharges. It produces a Tight pulse (see p.214) and a pale tongue (see p.216).

External Heat can penetrate the body of someone who lives or works in **Heat-Fire** an excessively hot environment – in an overly hot kitchen or bakery, for example. However, Heat and Fire most commonly originate from the Interior. They combine with external pathogenic factors such as Wind or Damp to produce additional symptoms of a Hot nature.
  Because of their strong Yang nature, Heat and Fire injure the Yin of the body. Apart from making one feel hot, Heat dries up the Body Fluids and causes thirst and a dry mouth. It can also cause burning pain.
  Fire displays these same characteristics, but is stronger and more 'solid' than Heat. Fire more commonly dries out the stools or causes constipation, and can make the Blood 'boil over' to cause bleeding. It has a greater effect on the Mind and more often results in mental agitation and insomnia. Its tendency to move upwards means that it can produce mouth ulcers and a bitter taste in the mouth. Both Heat and Fire produce a Rapid pulse and a red tongue.

Summer-Heat is a specific type of Heat invasion, only occurring as a **Summer-Heat** result of exposure to very hot weather, as in the case of sunstroke. Like Heat and Fire, it damages the Yin of the body, causing thirst, sweating, headache, and dark and scanty urine. If Summer-Heat invades the Heart Protector it can cause delirium and possibly unconsciousness. It produces a Rapid pulse and a red tongue.

Dryness is another external pathogenic factor which attacks the moist **Dryness** Yin of the body. The extreme dryness of certain natural and artificial environments can lead to dryness of the mouth, the tongue, the lips and the throat. The stools may become dry and urination dark and scanty.

Dampness   Dampness is heavy and cloying and so impedes the Yang of the body, especially the transformative function of the Spleen. Exposure to damp weather, wearing wet clothes and living in a damp environment may allow External Dampness to invade. External Dampness frequently penetrates the Channels and gathers in the joints to produce rheumatic symptoms. These are characterized by fixed dull aching, stiffness and swelling of the joints. External Dampness can also combine with Heat to generate a fever. The presence of External Dampness is indicated by a Full and Slippery pulse and a thick, sticky tongue coating.

Dampness can also be generated from within by a weakness in the function of the Spleen, involving the subsequent poor transformation and transportation of Body Fluids. This condition is often compounded by excessive consumption of Damp-producing foods such as dairy products and sugar. Internal Dampness is characterized by symptoms which arise much more slowly than External Dampness. It often causes tiredness and a heavy feeling in the limbs. It tends to sink to the Hara where it produces swelling and a sense of fullness. Internal Dampness collects in the chest to produce a feeling of congestion and commonly makes one feel heavy-headed. It is also evident in vaginal discharges and skin diseases involving pus. Internal Dampness may produce a Fine and Slippery pulse and a sticky tongue coating.

An important pathogenic factor which is similar to Dampness is Phlegm. Phlegm is also generated by an impairment of the body's ability to transform and transport Body Fluids. However, in the case of Phlegm production, this process involves not only the Spleen but the Kidneys and Lungs as well. Moreover, Phlegm is only produced internally, so is not an External cause of disease. Rather than sinking to the Hara, Phlegm tends to collect in the Stomach and rise to the Lungs, nose and throat. It can also 'mist the orifices' of the Heart and therefore cloud and confuse the Mind.

Both Dampness and Phlegm frequently combine with Heat and Cold, producing Damp-Cold and Damp-Heat, and Cold Phlegm and Hot Phlegm. Phlegm can also combine with Fire to form Phlegm-Fire. Dampness and Phlegm which are Cold in nature produce white or clear mucus and a white tongue coating; Damp-Heat, Hot Phlegm and Phlegm-Fire produce yellow mucus and a yellow tongue coating.

THE OTHER CAUSES OF DISEASE

The causes of disease which do not fit into the categories above are as follows:

- poor constitution
- poor dietary habits
- over-exertion
- excessive sexual activity
- trauma
- parasites and poisons
- Incorrect Treatment

Poor Constitution

An individual's constitutional strength is dependent on the health of their parents, particularly at the time of conception. This is the moment at which the Pre-Heaven Essence is formed from the fusion of the parental Essences. The foetal Essence becomes dependent on nourishment from the Mother. Her health during the period of gestation is thus another important factor in determining the strength of the child's constitution.

One's inherited (or Pre-Heaven) Essence is largely, though not completely, predetermined. It may be prematurely drained through overwork, excessive sexual activity and drug abuse; or it can be preserved and enhanced through special ways of self-development. Traditionally these include Tai Ji Quan, Qi Gong and Taoist forms of meditation and breathing exercises. Through building up one's reserve of Qi, a person with a relatively weak constitution may supplement their Essence with additional strength.

Poor Dietary Habits

Diet is of course a major cause of ill-health and plays a role in the development of almost all diseases. The subject of diet and health is a huge one but we can take a brief look at its most important aspects.

Dietary patterns in the West have two main problems: the over-consumption of foods of an animal origin; and the excessive influence of technology on agriculture and food production. The heavy reliance on meat and dairy products leads to a diet which is overly rich in fats. In addition, the livestock which produces these foods are fed hormones and antibiotics in order to enhance their profitability. The encroachment of technology upon the modern diet is further apparent in the heavy use of chemical fertilizers and pesticides as well as the widespread presence of chemical additives in food. All these influences heighten the possibility of degenerative disease.

Malnutrition is another serious problem, both in the Third World and the poorer areas of the West. It seriously weakens the Ki and Blood and results in Spleen deficiency, making it harder to absorb and make use of the little nourishment which is taken. Over-eating also weakens the Spleen and Stomach, and leads to 'Retention of Food', characterized by a bloated feeling in the stomach, belching, nausea and gastric reflux.

Regularly eating foods which are excessively Hot or Cold in energy is also detrimental to health. Too many cooling foods (such as salads, fruit, fruit juice, and ice cream) can injure the Yang of the Spleen. This impairs its transformative function (a function which requires warmth) and so leads to the accumulation of Dampness and Phlegm. Abdominal swelling and diarrhoea commonly result.

Foods which are very Hot in nature include beef, pork, alcohol and spicy food. Eaten in excess, they can create symptoms of Heat in the Liver or Stomach. These include a burning pain in the stomach and a bitter taste in the mouth. Oily, fried and greasy foods will again lead to a build-up of Dampness and Phlegm, impairing in particular the function of the Spleen. Phlegm will be evident in congested sinuses and a thick tongue coating.

Generally speaking, it is considered that a healthy diet should include cereal grains and their products, vegetables, beans, fruits, seeds and nuts. Unless one is vegetarian, eating fish and white meat is preferable to the frequent consumption of red meat. Also advisable is the moderate use of cold-pressed oils (N.B. cold-pressed oils should not be used for cooking at high temperatures) and natural, unrefined sweeteners. Medicinal diets must always be based on an accurate assessment of the patient's needs.

Those who are predominantly Yang-deficient will require a greater degree of warming foods such as cereal grains and cooked vegetables in their diet. They will do well to make use of items such as ginger and garlic in their cooking, both of which strengthen the body's Yang functions. Those patients who are predominantly Yin-deficient will need a higher proportion of cooling and moistening foods, such as lightly-cooked or raw vegetables and fruit. Special foods to tonify the Yin include pumpkin and fruits in general.

Food should always be eaten in a calm and settled state. Eating when upset or worried, eating in a hurry, or eating and working at the same time will deplete the Stomach and Spleen and impair digestion.

Over-Exertion Mental and physical over-exertion is a frequent cause of health problems in the West. Adequate rest is always necessary to replenish one's reserve of Ki. Insufficient rest over a number of months or years will mean that the body will have to draw on the Essence for additional strength. This will ultimately lead to a depletion of the Essence and to a weakening of the constitution.

Physical overwork puts a particular strain on the Spleen because it dominates the muscles. Repetitive use of certain muscles may cause localized Ki or Blood stagnation. Shiatsu therapy can do much to alleviate these conditions because of the effect it has on promoting circulation and improving muscle tone. An associated form of physical over-exertion is to found in people who engage in irregular and exhausting exercise, thus injuring Ki. On the other hand, a lack of exercise will lead to stagnation of Ki.

Because the Spleen houses Thought, it is easily weakened by excessive mental activity. Mental overwork also tends to consume the Yin of the body and therefore depletes the Stomach and Kidneys.

Excessive sexual activity has in the East traditionally been viewed as depleting to one's vital energy. The sexual energies of both men and women are derived from the Kidney-Essence. The body draws on the Essence in order to achieve ejaculation and orgasm. When there is insufficient time allowed between sexual activity for the replenishment of the Essence, and it outstrips one's reserve, a deficiency of Essence will ensue.

Excessive Sexual Activity

What is considered excessive sexual activity therefore depends upon the strength of one's Essence. The Essence reaches a peak in the early twenties and then begins to decline slowly. It also varies according to the individual: because some people have a strong constitution, they can engage in a relatively greater degree of sexual activity without depleting their Essence.

There is also a distinction to be made between men and women. Male sexual energy is more closely related to the Essence than female sexual energy. Ejaculation for men therefore represents a greater loss of Essence than orgasm for women. However, women also lose Essence through the process of childbirth, and may become deficient when the birth of one child is too quickly followed by another.

Strengthening the sexual function and replenishing the Essence requires treatment of the Kidneys, the basis of these energies. Kidney-Yang is responsible for mobilizing the Essence, especially in men; a deficiency will lead to impotence and premature ejaculation. Kidney-Essence and Kidney-Yin are especially important for the nourishment of the Uterus; their deficiency may cause infertility.

Trauma refers to physical accidents such as broken bones and bruising. Traumas result in localized stagnation of Ki, and stagnation of Blood if they are serious. Occasionally they cause long-term stagnation of Ki or Blood, especially when combined with other causes of disease such as External Dampness. External factors more easily penetrate into areas of the body weakened by a previous trauma and complicate an existing problem.

Trauma

Parasites – in the form of worms – and poisons are causes of disease which most frequently affect children. Clearly, they are problems which are not easily treated through Shiatsu.

Parasites and Poisons

The more invasive the type of treatment, the bigger the potential disaster from incorrect treatment. Therefore wrong surgery or wrong oral medicines or herbs can be more damaging than shiatsu treatment based on incorrect diagnosis.

Incorrect Treatment

Chapter 10

The Five Elements

INTRODUCTION

The Five Elements – Water, Wood, Fire, Earth and Metal – are an important aspect of Traditional Oriental Medicine. As an energetic system calling for intuitive insight and logic, it provides the Shiatsu practitioner with a tool to understand their patient physically, psychologically and spiritually. There are a number of points to grasp about the Five Elements before exploring them in detail individually.

It is significant that the Five Elements consist of five energetic stages rather than four, as in the Western tradition of Fire, Earth, Air and Water. Esoteric philosophers have understood the number five to symbolize dynamic interchange, and thus to represent Nature. This is precisely how the Five Elements are best understood: as stages of transformation which interconnect on every level of the natural world and the human microcosm of the bodymind.

Seeing the Five Elements as phases of a process rather than fixed representations of matter is supported by the literal meaning of the Chinese term for the 'Five Phases': *wu xing*. *Wu* means 'five', and *xing* means 'walk' or 'move'. The Five Elements express the 'five movements' of the Universe. As emblems of Nature they relate to a multitude of phenomena (season, colour, emotion and so on), but express the energetic quality of those phenomena as if they were different 'movements' of a whole. From this viewpoint, the Five Elements can be seen as an extrapolation of the movements of Yin and Yang (see Fig. 10.1).

THE CREATION CYCLE

Let us look at how the Five Elements embody the energetic stages of Yin/Yang. The Water Element possesses the Yin quality of life at rest; energy which is in a floating state (as in Winter). Wood gives this potential state the Yang qualities of direction and growth; energy rising (as in Spring). Growth leads to self-awareness, central to the Fire Element; energy expanding and reaching a peak (as in Summer). Earth gives this awareness bodily form, balancing it with Yin; energy descending earthwards (as in Late Summer). Metal completes the cycle through exchanging the outworn for the new; energy gathering to be dispersed (as in Autumn). Metal is Yin in function because it acts as a stable meeting point. Each stage generates and is the 'Mother' of the next, its 'Child'.

Since the Five Phases theory was first systematized around 300 BC, this sequential order of the Elements, called the *Shen* or 'Creation' Cycle, underwent many changes, and may not in reality be fixed. The modern order outlined here, however, is logical. It is seen at work in Nature in the way that Water nourishes Wood; Wood burns to make Fire; the ashes of Fire decompose into Earth; Earth contains the ores of Metal; and Metal melts into 'Water' (the liquid state).

A SUMMARY OF THE ELEMENTS

The Water Element is associated with night-time and with rest. It provides us with the instinct for survival and the emotion of Fear, as well as the urge to procreate. It is the source of Will (*Zhi*) in the

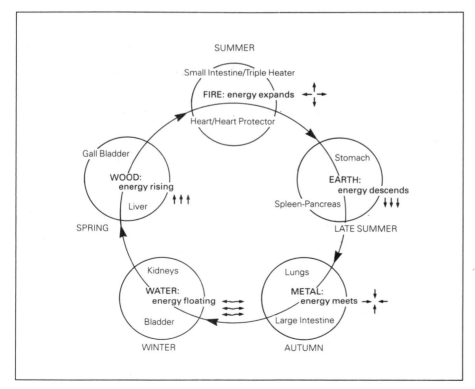

Fig. 10.1: Creation cycle

bodymind, and provides it with endurance. Water relates to the Yin (Zang) Organ of the Kidneys, which house the Essence (*Jing*), the basis of our constitutional strength. Its coupled Yang (Fu) Organ, also belonging to Water, is the Bladder. A person with a predominance of the Water Element will have a blue tinge to the colour of their face, a groaning sound in their voice, and a slight putrid odour (discernible near the chest or back). They may be slightly timid in character, or inwardly insecure.

The Wood Element is associated with the morning and with initiating action. It provides the ability to plan, control and assert, and affords the capacity for Anger. Wood relates to the Yin (Zang) Organ of the Liver, which houses the Ethereal Soul (*Hun*). The Ethereal Soul oversees our individual evolution, and is the source of hope and vision. The Yang (Fu) Organ which belongs to the Wood Element is the Gall Bladder, the seat of initiative. A person with a predominance of Wood energy will have a green tinge to the colour of their face, a slight shouting or clipped quality to the sound of their voice, and a faint rancid odour. They tend to be authoritative, well-organized and frequently irritable.

The Fire Element is associated with noon and activity at its peak. It represents our self-identity and urge to celebrate, bestowing the capacity for Joy and Love. Fire relates to the Yin Organ of the Heart, which houses the Mind (*Shen*). The Mind is the foundation of consciousness and the origin of thought and emotion. It is the most rarefied Ki of all. The Fire Element also encompasses the Organs of the Small Intestines, the Heart Protector and the Triple Heater. A person with a predominance of Fire energy will have a red tinge to the colour of their face, a laughing or tremulous quality to the sound of their voice, and a faint scorched odour. They are usually sensitive, excitable or emotionally changeable in nature.

The Earth Element is associated with the late afternoon and with a decrease in activity. It produces the ability to concentrate and analyse, granting the capacity for Pensiveness. Earth relates to the Yin Organ of the Spleen, which houses Thought (*Yi*). Thought provides the Mind with a logical process, just as the Spleen subjects food to a digestive process. Its coupled Yang Organ is the Stomach, the seat of our ability to listen and absorb. A person with a predominance of Earth energy will have a yellow tinge to the colour of their face, a singing quality to the sound of their voice, and a faintly sweet, or fragrant odour. They are often sympathetic listeners and have a tendency to worry.

The Metal Element is associated with the evening and a balance between activity and rest. It provides us with a sense of boundary across which we can take in and let go. Connected to the process of 'letting go' is the emotion of the Metal Element: that of Grief. Metal relates to the Yin Organ of the Lungs, which houses the Corporeal Soul (*P'o*). The Corporeal Soul gives us our 'animal' vitality and inherent optimism; when it is stricken we become despondent. The associated Yang Organ of the Metal Element is the Large Intestines. A person with a predominance of Metal energy will have a white tinge to the colour of their face, a subtle weeping quality to the sound of their voice, and a faint rotten odour. Although they can easily feel 'invaded', they quickly become melancholic if they 'lose touch' with those important to them.

The Control Cycle

A second set of relationships exist between alternate Elements of the Shen Cycle. In its normal clockwise movement, this interaction is known as the *Ko*, or 'Control', Cycle. The Ko Cycle may be expressed through the imagery of Nature as follows: Wood is cut by Metal; Metal is melted by Fire; Fire is extinguished by Water; Water is channelled by Earth; and Earth is penetrated by Wood (see Fig. 10.2).

To illustrate this 'control': the Water Element, through providing the 'Bone Marrow' that fills the brain, anchors the Mind of the Fire Element, whose underlying nature is to expand. The expansive radiance of the Self found in Fire controls Metal's tendency to concentrate and refine. Metal controls Wood through providing it with the sense of boundary and structure it needs to maintain order. The free-flow of energy in Wood ensures that Earth's transformative processes are smooth and harmoniously ordered. Finally, Earth harnesses the primordial power of Water by channelling it into physical processes.

The Shen and Ko cycles reflect two different 'movements' of the Five Elements. The Shen Cycle relationships are relatively more Yin: they are mutually nourishing and unifying. Ko Cycle interaction is relatively

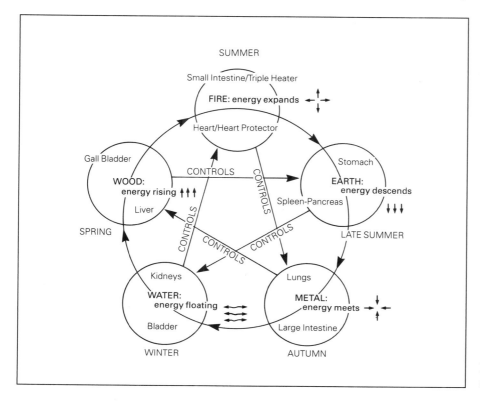

Fig. 10.2: Control cycle

more Yang: it reflects the antagonistic qualities of the Elements. Here they set mutual limits and so give each other structure, producing a cycle of 'control'.

THE FIVE ELEMENTS IN SHIATSU

The Five Elements serve the Shiatsu practitioner in three interconnected ways: they can enhance accurate physical diagnosis; provide a comprehensive model for understanding and treating the patient on an emotional level; and deepen philosophical insight.

On a level of physical diagnosis, they highlight the functions of the Organs they are associated with, making their dysfunctions clearer. They are not, however, an important means of understanding disease in Oriental Medicine, and are secondary to a thorough grasp of the Theory of the Organs (the *Zangfu*). It was only relatively recently in the history of Chinese Medicine, in the Song Dynasty (960–1279 AD), that the interactions of the Five Elements were commonly employed in the diagnosis and treatment of illness. Nevertheless, they provide a flexible yet revealing model for understanding the patient psychologically, and can lead the attentive practitioner to a deep insight into the Internal cause of a disease.

No one is in a state of perfect harmony: we all have certain psychological tendencies which, when over- or under-activated, concentrate emotional energy in certain Elements and not others. Each of the five basic 'attitudes' (or *zhi*) – Fear (Water), Anger (Wood), Joy (Fire), Pensiveness (Earth) and Grief (Metal) – are necessary to complete our character. But when we get 'stuck' in one or two of these 'attitudes' they can intensify into 'passions' (*qing*) and so dominate the psyche.

For example, we have seen from our observations of the Ko Cycle that the Water Element 'controls' Fire, partly through 'rooting' the mind. If the Water Element becomes afflicted, both physically and psychologically, through over-work and mental strain, the Kidneys (Water) will fail to provide a secure foundation for the Heart (Fire). This allows the Mind to become over-excited and nervous. When coupled with a vague sense of fear precipitated by a weakened Water Element, feelings of anxiety may result.

Understanding the causation of anxiety from this perspective allows the Shiatsu practitioner to formulate an appropriate and effective treatment strategy. In this particular case, they should consider tonifying the Channels and associated areas of the Kidneys, as well as dispersing those of the Heart. Particular emphasis could be given to treatment of the following Tsubos: Kidney-6 (tonifies Kidney Yin and calms the Mind); Bladder-23 (strengthens Ki of Kidneys); Directing Vessel-4 (supports firm foundation of the Kidneys and roots the Mind); Heart-7 and Directing Vessel-15 (both calm the Heart and the Mind).

The Five Elements are therefore of great practical value in Shiatsu.

They can, at the same time, be of spiritual value to the natural healer. As a dynamic model of wholeness, they can allow us to look at our own life and assess, in a non-judgemental spirit, the relative balance of its different parts. For example, we may ask ourselves how we touch our deepest core and self-renew (Water)? Whether we have a harmonious sense of achievement in life, being neither driven nor without vision (Wood)? Can we allow ourselves to love, and so be essentially self-fulfilled (Fire)? Do we truly listen to life, integrate experience and allow it to change us (Earth)? Finally, do we feel 'connected' to others, neither cut-off or impinged upon (Metal)?

As a tool of meditation we can employ the Five Elements on a more subtle level through visualizing those Elements in which we may feel particularly challenged. For example, to cultivate self-confidence and easy authority (Wood), we may visualize the rooted sturdiness of a tree, its limbs of strength reaching upwards. To relieve melancholy and revive the brilliance of inner Ki (Metal), we can visualize the diamond or crystal and its vibrant power to receive, refract and radiate, simultaneously, always in the present moment.

Now we are ready to explore each of the Five Elements and their associated Organs in detail.

Chapter 11

Water: The Kidneys and Bladder

The natural point of departure for an in-depth discussion of the Five Elements and their associated Yin and Yang Organs begins with the Water Element. This is because Water is representative of life's beginning. As Lao Tzu says in the Tao Te Ching: 'Water gives life to the ten thousand things and does not strive.'

In the world's oldest creation myth, the ancient Sumerians ascribed the creative principle to the sea. The same hieroglyph also represented both the Goddess of Water and human sperm. To the Chinese, too, the Water Element symbolized the source of life, containing within itself life's many possible creations.

In the body, this originating aspect of the Water Element is reflected in the Original Ki and its substantial basis, the Essence (or *Jing*, both of which are controlled by the Kidneys. The Kidneys are the Yin Organ of the Water Element; the Bladder its Yang Organ. The Essence forms the 'core' of the bodymind and could be said, in scientific terms, to contain the genetic material needed for conception and new life.

The Source of Life provides the will-to-be and will-to-create: thus it is the Kidneys which house the Will (or *Zhi*) of the bodymind. The Will provides the instinct for survival and drive to procreate. It is when the Will is threatened in some way that fear emerges within the psyche. When the Will is strong we are invested with self-confidence and an innate trust in what life will bring. The energetic centre of the Will is located deep in the Hara, at the 'Gate of Vitality', the source of our strength and stability.

The season of Water is Winter, when the energy of the Earth is in a dormant, floating state, and when the potential plant is but a seed, waiting for the warmth of Spring. The nature of the Water Element may be further explored and more clearly understood through an analysis of the functions of its associated Yin organ, the Kidneys.

THE FUNCTIONS OF THE KIDNEYS

Store the Essence   The first function of the Kidneys is to store the Essence which in turn governs the processes of birth, growth, reproduction and development. We have already looked at the Essence in some detail and have seen that it is closely related to the Kidneys. The Kidneys host and sustain the Essence, and together they ensure that we develop according to an original 'plan'. This plan is unique to each individual, and is contained in the genetic code formed at conception. It is the work of the Kidney Essence to sustain this plan against a variety of environmental and pathogenic influences. It thus ensures the integrity and cohesion of the individual.

The Essence manifests itself over time through the process of physical and mental growth. Problems relating to the Essence may result in retarded growth or premature aging. Because the Essence provides the basis for sexual development, infertility or a lack of sexual vitality can also occur.

A natural and harmonious decline is as much an expression of a healthy Essence as is normal growth and development in children. If one expresses one's willpower wisely, the Essence is well preserved and diminishes slowly. The wise person adapts to its decline and makes perfect use of the Essence they have, thus maintaining vitality.

Produce the Marrow

The second function of the Kidneys, closely related to the first, is that they 'produce the Marrow, fill up the brain and control the bones'. Just as they provide, through the Essence, the genetic structure of the body, so they provide it with physical structure in the form of the bones and teeth. However, the Oriental concept of the Marrow includes not only the bone-marrow, but the brain, nerves and spinal cord as well. The Marrow is part of the Essence and therefore fundamentally Yin in nature. Forming the physical basis of the nervous system it hosts its energetic Yang polarity, the Mind (or Shen).

Govern Water

The third main function of the Kidneys is directly associated with their Western physiological function; namely, that the Kidneys govern Water in the body. The Kidneys have a close relationship with the Lower Heater, which includes the entire lower abdomen below the level of the umbilicus. The organs in this area are often compared to a 'drainage ditch', as they are responsible for the excretion of impure Body Fluids. The Kidneys may be thought of as a 'gate' which opens and closes to control this flow of fluids. When Kidney-Yang is deficient, the gate is too open, leading to copious, clear urination. When Kidney-Yin is deficient, the gate is too closed, leading to scanty, dark urination.

Control the Reception of Ki

This function of the Kidneys highlights their close relationship with the Lungs. The Kidneys grasp and anchor the Ki descended by the Lungs following inhalation. If the Kidney-Yang becomes deficient, and this function weakens, Ki will become trapped in the chest and asthma may develop.

Open into the Ears   The Kidneys open into the ears, because the ears depend upon sustenance from the Essence to function well. Problems related to hearing, such as tinnitus (ringing in the ears) may be related to Kidney weakness.

Manifest on the Hair   Finally, the Kidneys manifest on the hair, which, like the ears, depends upon the Essence for normal growth. Abundant, shining hair reflects a vital Kidney-Essence; hair which is thin, brittle and greying may indicate that the Essence is weakening.

THE FUNCTIONS OF THE BLADDER

The role of the Bladder in 'The Yellow Emperor's Classic' is compared to that of 'a district official, it stores the fluids so that they can be excreted by its action of Ki transformation'. The function of the Bladder, therefore, is the transformation of fluids under the action of Ki supplied by the Kidney-Yang. It receives the impure fluids from the Small Intestines and transforms them into urine for storage and subsequent excretion.

SHIATSU TREATMENT OF THE KIDNEYS

In Shiatsu treatment, the Kidneys will often require tonification due to the key supportive role they play in relation to the other major Yin organs. First, the Kidney-Yin is vital for the nourishment of the Liver (Water feeds Wood). It also prevents the Liver from over-heating (due to the Liver's Yang nature and wide array of functions). The Kidney-Yang plays a crucial role in supporting the transformative action of the Spleen-Yang, providing it with the Fire necessary for digestion. The Heart relies on both the Kidney-Yang for force and the Kidney-Yin for nourishment; the Kidney-Yin also helps to anchor the Mind. Again, the Lungs rely on the Kidneys to 'grasp the Ki' derived from breathing. It is understandable, therefore, that the Kidneys are considered to be 'the root of Yin and Yang'.

Signs and symptoms common to Kidney problems in general include lower-back pain, dark rings under the eyes, a groaning sound in the voice, and feelings of insecurity, anxiety or fear.

Treatment of Kidney-Essence Deficiency   In the Shiatsu clinic the most common type of patient requiring strengthening of the Essence is the elderly person with problems such as Osteoporosis, Osteoarthritis, loss of memory, loss of hair and teeth, and chronic fatigue. Because Ki and Blood deficiency are commonly involved, the tongue and face are likely to be a dull, pale colour, and the pulse Empty. The Kidney Channel will generally be Kyo in condition. However, always tonify the *most* Kyo Channel, which could in practice, be *any* other channel.

The main Tsubos for tonifying the Essence are Kidney-3 and Directing Vessel-4. The Tsubo Bladder-23 (Kidney Yu Point) will support the Essence through strengthening the Kidneys. Tonification of Gall Bladder-39 is called for in cases of Osteoporosis, as it tonifies the Bone Marrow. The Tsubo Bladder-11 (Gathering Point for the Bones) also helps to strenthen the bones.

Treatment of Kidney-Yin Deficiency

It is important to remember that the Kidneys are the body's source of Yin (moisture, nourishment and cooling). Kidney-Yin deficiency is apparent when signs of Kidney weakness such as lower-back pain combine with those of deficient Yin. Signs of Yin deficiency include hot hands and feet, dry mouth and sweating at night, and dark, scanty urine. The pulse will be Empty at a deep level (see p.213). The tongue will be red and possibly cracked, peeled or without a coating (see p.215).

Kidney-Yin may be tonified through the sustained holding of the lower Hara and treatment of the Bladder Channel in the lower back. Tonify the Tsubos Kidney-6 and -3, Directing Vessel-4 and Spleen-6, all of which tonify Kidney-Yin.

(See Case Study Example No. 2 on p.225.)

Treatment of Kidney-Yang Deficiency

The Kidneys are closely related to the 'Gate of Vitality' and are the source of the body's Yang (i.e. warmth and motive force). A weakness of Kidney-Yang will directly affect the Yang of the entire body. Signs of Kidney-Yang deficiency include lethargy, pallor, coldness in the back and legs, weakness and oedema of the legs, loose stools and copious, clear urination. The pulse will be Empty and the tongue swollen and pale.

Kidney-Yang may be strengthened through the deep tonification of the lower Hara and treatment of the Bladder Channel in the lower back. Tsubos which strengthen Kidney-Yang include Bladder-23, Directing Vessel-4 and -6, and Kidney-3 and -7.

When weakness of Kidney-Yang leads to an impairment in the Kidney function of grasping the Ki, Lung-7 and Kidney-6 may be treated simultaneously. These two Tsubos in combination open the Directing Vessel, which, among other things, helps the Lungs and Kidneys to communicate. This may also be achieved by holding, with light finger pressure, both Directing Vessel-6 and -17, the lower and upper 'Sea of Ki' points (see Fig. 11.1).

THE SPIRIT OF WATER

Let us take a final look at the role of the Water Element in the bodymind. We have seen how Water is the source of our life-force and Will. When this is challenged and our survival is threatened we experience fear. However, a vague, subconscious fear may arise in patterns of Kidney disharmony, and manifest as insecurity, anxiety and mistrust. Treating the Kidneys with Shiatsu will help not only to alleviate problems such as lower-back pain, but will improve emotional health as well.

The tonification of Tsubo Bladder-52 ('Will Power Room') is especially good for restoring confidence and purpose. Tonifying the Kidney Channel in the chest restores the Will when there is timidity and a feeling of being overwhelmed.

According to Ted Kaptchuk,[1] the Water Element preserves the 'Virtue' (or 'Destiny') of Wisdom. It requires Wisdom to direct creatively the Will, as well as to harness and sustain it. It requires Wisdom, too, to cast aside fear when the Will is seriously challenged. To have an attitude which is neither over-powering nor wilful, or indeed easily overcome, ensures a wise and strong will-power.

This idea is crucial to good Shiatsu. The wise practitioner will work from their source, from their Hara. They will 'listen' to the patient's body and naturally find the right depth and strength of treatment. A strong and open Hara, one of the essentials of competent Shiatsu, is a sign of a healthy Water Element: they are ultimately one and the same.

The Water Element is also linked to technical ability – another essential ingredient of Shiatsu. The Kidneys are responsible for 'the power that is the underpinning of life from its beginning. This force or power is expressed with "skill" and "cleverness". with "know-how".'[2]

NOTES

1. Ted Kaptchuk, *The Way of the Spirit*, a public lecture held in London, November 1989.
2. Claude Larre, Jean Schatz and Elisabeth Rochat de la Vallee, *Survey of Traditional Chinese Medicine*, translated by Sarah Elizabeth Stang, Institut Ricci, Paris, and Traditional Acupuncture Institute, U.S.A., 1986, p.176.

Chapter 12

Wood: The Liver and Gall Bladder

As we have seen from our study of the Creation Cycle of the Five Elements, the raw force of Water yields to the organizing phase of Wood. The Wood Element does more than simply order and channel the drive of the Water Element, it lends it vision and gives it aspiration. Wood represents the 'giving of images'. Whereas Water is the seed, the symbol of potential growth, Wood is the shoot, and represents actual growth. The Wood Element is often called 'Tree-Phase', and encapsulates the rising energy of Spring-time.

The Yin Organ of the Wood Element, the Liver, is said in 'The Yellow Emperor's Classic' to be 'like an army's General from whom the strategy is derived'. The Liver harnesses the power of the bodymind and gives it a sense of direction. It ensures that our vital forces flow in harmony and according to plan. It is thus known as the 'Strategic Planner' among the twelve Organs, and is the source of our authority and decisiveness.

The Liver is assisted in this capacity by its paired Yang organ, the Gall Bladder, 'the upright Official that takes decisions'. The role of the Gall Bladder as 'decision-maker' is derived from its 'courageous' nature. The Gall Bladder takes the drive inherent in the Water Element and gives it decisiveness and action. It thus contributes to our courage and initiative.

The role of the Gall Bladder contrasts with the decision-making ability of the Small Intestines, which is based on its analytical power to 'separate the pure from the impure'. Rather than being a source of decisiveness as such, the Small Intestines help determine our clarity of mind.

THE FUNCTIONS OF THE LIVER

Smoothes the Flow of Ki
The channelling action of the Wood Element is seen at work in the Liver's function of ensuring the smooth flow of Ki. This function is of vital importance to every area of the bodymind. If it fails, the mind becomes tense and bodily processes obstructed.

The stagnation and build-up of Ki are closely associated with frustration or depression. These emotions can both cause and result from Ki stagnation. We are more likely to get frustrated or depressed when the plans and visions of the Wood Element are thwarted. Getting angry also reflects a blockage of Ki, and sometimes helps release it. Anger which turns inwards appears in muted forms such as brooding resentment or deep depression. Longstanding emotions of a repressed nature can also generate Fire in the body.

Digestive problems are frequently caused by Ki stagnation due to Liver disharmony. These involve an array of symptoms reflecting a disruption of normal energy flow in the Stomach and Spleen. In terms of the Five Elements, Wood 'invades' Earth along the Control Cycle. The symptoms include indigestion, nausea, bloating, flatulence and sometimes epigastric pain.

The normal direction of Stomach-Ki is downwards: when this is disrupted there are signs of so-called 'rebellious Ki'; energy moves upwards in the form of belching, gastric reflux ('heartburn') and vomiting. The normal direction of Spleen-Ki is upwards: when this is obstructed there are loose stools, diarrhoea and possibly prolapse.

Stagnant Liver-Ki can also obstruct the flow of bile, leading to poor digestion of fats, and in some cases jaundice. Feelings of tightness or oppression in the chest, of a lump in the throat and of distension of the breasts frequently reflect stagnation of Liver-Ki. Constipation may also have its root in this problem. General signs of stagnant Liver-Ki include a Wiry pulse, a purple tongue, rigidity of movement and chronic stiffness.

Stores the Blood

The second major function of the Liver is that it stores the Blood. This function seems simple in nature but effects the body in a number of ways. The Liver regulates the amount of Blood in circulation in accordance with levels of physical activity. During rest a large proportion of Blood flows to the Liver to be stored; when the body is active again, it returns to general circulation. This function ensures that the body receives adequate amounts of nourishment and energy.

If it becomes impaired and the Liver fails to store the Blood properly, Blood Deficiency may develop, producing such signs as fatigue, pallor, dizziness, dry skin, brittle nails and 'floaters' (spots) in the field of vision. The pulse will be Choppy or Thready and the tongue dull-pale and dry.

Controls the Sinews

The third function of the Liver is that it controls the sinews, i.e. the tendons, the ligaments and muscular action. Properly nourished by the Liver-Blood, the sinews will contract and relax in a way that ensures the smooth movement of the joints and ease of muscular action. When Liver-Blood is deficient, the tendons are more likely to become stiff, causing joint immobility and weakness in the limbs. More serious Liver disharmonies may lead to tetany and tremors involving the tendons.

Manifests in the Nails

The nails depend, like the sinews with which they are associated, on the nourishment of Liver-Blood. Signs of deficiency of Liver-Blood include nails which have become indented, cracked and dry.

Opens into the Eyes

Liver-Blood nourishes and maintains the eyes. Liver-Blood that is deficient may lead to dry and gritty eyes, poor vision and the presence of spots or 'floaters'. When there is excess Heat in the Liver the eyes often feel burning or painful. It should be remembered, however, that many of the Organs influence the condition of the eyes, so that not all eye problems are caused by the Liver.

The Liver Yu point, Bladder-18, may be treated for all eye problems. The Tsubo Gall-Bladder-37 (named 'Brightness') 'brightens the eyes'. Kidney-6 benefits the vision through nourishing the eyes.

THE FUNCTIONS OF THE GALL BLADDER

The functions of the Gall Bladder are relatively few and simple. We have already seen how the Gall Bladder plays an important role in decision-making and initiative. A person who pushes themself too hard will put particular strain on their Gall Bladder.

Its main physical function is the same as that of Western Medicine, the storage and excretion of bile. The efficiency with which this function operates is again dependent on the smooth flow of Ki. In turn, the health of the Gall Bladder influences the Liver's ability to regulate the Ki. The condition of these paired Organs is always closely connected.

SHIATSU TREATMENT OF THE LIVER AND GALL BLADDER

Treatment of Stagnant Liver/Gall Bladder Ki

Stagnant Ki requires moving (i.e. dispersing): because to over-tonify the body of a person with stagnant Ki may exacerbate their condition. Happily, it is difficult to over-tonify with Shiatsu; it is more easily done with Acupuncture or Herbal Medicine.

When there is Ki stagnation, the Liver and Gall Bladder Channels will commonly present as Jitsu in condition. The Liver may also cause Ki stagnation in other Organs, especially the Stomach, Spleen, Heart, Heart Protector and Large Intestines, producing a Jitsu condition in these Channels as well. A variety of stretching techniques should be employed to move the Ki, with emphasis on opening the Gall Bladder Channel in the Side Position.

The main Tsubos to treat for stagnant Ki are Gall Bladder-34 and

Liver-3. Both Tsubos are called for when stagnant Liver-Ki affects the epigastrium and abdomen, causing problems such as nausea, indigestion and abdominal distension and pain. Gall Bladder-34 is especially important to treat in most cases of constipation. Both Tsubos should also be treated when there are muscular cramps and spasms in the body. Because Liver-3 has a strong calming action on the Liver, it is excellent for treatment of headaches.

Gall-Bladder-41 is another Tsubo which may be used for headaches due to stagnant Liver-Ki; it can also be dispersed to relieve breast pain and distension. The Tsubos Liver-13 and -14, both located under the rib cage, move the Liver-Ki when it disrupts the digestion. Both Tsubos help to harmonize Wood and Earth: Liver-13 is more effective for stagnant Liver-Ki 'invading' the Spleen; Liver-14 is more important for stagnant Liver-Ki 'invading' the Stomach. Among the many actions of the Tsubo Spleen-6 is its ability to smooth the Liver-Ki, especially in the Lower Heater. Finally, Heart Protector-6 is excellent for stagnant Ki in the chest, resulting in a sense of constriction or oppression.

Treatment of Liver-Blood Deficiency

Because the Liver stores the Blood, a deficiency of Blood will often create a Kyo condition of the Liver Channel, along with those of the Spleen and Kidney but tonify whichever Channel actually presents itself as the *most* Kyo Channel. It is also very useful to treat specific points which tonify Blood. As the Yu points have a powerful tonifying effect, treat Tsubos Bladder-18 (Liver Yu Point), Bladder-20 (Spleen Yu Point) and Bladder-23 (Kidney Yu Point). Applying moxibustion to the Yu Point of the Blood, Bladder-17, as well as Directing Vessel-4, will also strengthen Blood. Finally, tonifying Stomach-36 tonifies the Blood through increasing the digestive power.

Gynaecological Aspects of Liver-Blood

The Liver's function of storing Blood has a very strong relationship with both the normal and abnormal functioning of the female gynaecological system. If the Liver-Blood is deficient, it may well affect menstruation, causing amenorrhoea (a lack of periods). It is also possible for the Liver to transmit Heat into the Blood, making the Blood 'boil over' and cause menorrhagia (excessive menstrual bleeding) as well as metrorrhagia (bleeding between periods). The very close link between the Liver and menstruation also means that stagnant Liver-Ki often results in pre-menstrual tension and menstrual pain. The presence of dark clots in menstrual blood is a sign that Ki-Stagnation has led to Blood-Stagnation.

When periods are scanty or absent altogether in a woman with other signs of Blood Deficiency, treat them according to the same principles as those for Liver-Blood Deficiency (mentioned above), adding some sustained Hara work, especially where the abdomen is Kyo in condition.

In order to cool the Blood in cases of excessive menstruation or abnormal bleeding, one may disperse the Tsubos Liver-2 and Spleen-10.

The Liver Yu Point, Bladder-18, may be treated to regulate the Blood.

Bladder-18 is also called for when there is severe menstrual pain and the presence of clots due to Ki and Blood Stagnation. The Liver and Gall Bladder Channels in this instance will tend to be Jitsu in condition and should be dispersed. Disperse the Tsubos Gall Bladder-34, Liver-3 and Directing Vessel-6 to move Ki and Blood in the Hara.

Treatment of Liver-Yang Rising

In the Creation Cycle of the Five Elements, Water nourishes Wood. This can be seen at work in the fact that the Kidney-Yin moistens and nourishes the Liver. When a deficiency of Kidney-Yin leads to a depletion of Liver-Yin, the Yang of the Liver is allowed to predominate over the Yin. Unchecked by descending Yin, its natural tendency is to rise, causing symptoms which affect the head.

Headaches often occur, affecting the eyes and the sides of the head, the mouth and throat may become dry, and there may be dizziness and tinnitus (ringing in the ears). The patient may report a difficulty in sleeping and controlling their temper; they will often be irritable and angry. The pulse will be Wiry and the tongue red (especially along the sides). These symptoms may be coupled with those of Kidney-Yin deficiency, including lower back pain, night sweating and hot hands and feet.

It is common in this instance to find that the Liver and Gall Bladder Channels are Jitsu in condition and the Kidney Channel is Kyo. If so, disperse the Liver and Gall Bladder Channels and tonify that of the Kidney. In the case of frequent headaches, be sure to include techniques to release the neck and ease the shoulders and temporal areas of the head. The most important Tsubo to sedate Liver-Yang is Liver-3. Gall Bladder-20 is called for in the case of frequent headaches and problems affecting the eyes. Triple Heater-5 may be dispersed in the case of headaches on the sides of the head. To strengthen Kidney-Yin, tonify the Tsubos Kidney-6 and -3, Directing Vessel-4 and Spleen-6.

(See Case Study Example No. 2 on p.225.)

Treatment of Liver-Fire

Fire in the Liver manifests most of the same signs and symptoms as Liver-Yang rising, but does not result from Kidney-Yin deficiency. Liver-Fire is an Excess pattern, whereas Liver-Yang rising is a pattern which involves both Empty and Excess conditions. Both patterns usually result from prolonged feelings of anger and frustration, although the emotions which generate Liver-Fire are either more extreme or repressed. Also, Liver-Fire is more often associated with the excessive intake of red meat, fatty foods and alcohol.

Liver-Fire can be distinguished from Liver-Yang rising in that it commonly produces a red face, red eyes, a bitter taste in the mouth and constipation. The pulse will be Full and Rapid; the tongue red with a yellow coating.

Liver-Fire will again tend to produce a Jitsu condition of the Liver and Gall Bladder Channels. Check the Heart and Heart Protector Channels as well; Fire is often transmitted from the Liver to the chest. Disperse the Liver and Gall Bladder Channels and the Tsubos Liver-2 and Gall Bladder-20, both of which sedate Liver-Fire.

Treatment of Liver-Wind

A deficiency of Liver-Blood or Liver-Yin, or a condition of extreme Liver-Heat, can on rare occasions give rise to a serious disharmony known as Internal Wind. Internal Wind should not be confused with External Wind: the two are fundamentally different. Internal Wind is generated by the Liver from within, and is characterized by dizziness and vertigo, tremor, rigidity, paralysis and convulsions.

Check whether the Liver Channel is Kyo or Jitsu in condition and treat accordingly. The main Tsubos to disperse Internal Wind are Liver-3, Gall Bladder-20 and Governing Vessel-16 and -20.

THE SPIRIT OF WOOD

A final, more subtle function of the Liver is that it houses the Ethereal Soul (or *Hun*). The Ethereal Soul is the part of the bodymind considered to survive after death and return to the world of immaterial existence. When properly rooted by the Yin and Blood, it provides us with our visionary capacity, which is intrinsic to the Wood Element; e.g. the Liver opens into the eyes.

If it becomes divorced from its physical 'home' the Ethereal Soul loses touch with its life's purpose and wanders aimlessly, divorced from reality. We lose our sense of living in the present. The bodymind compensates for this by erecting mental structures to mask a lack of inner meaning. But ultimately the rigidity which this encourages only creates frustration and intolerance. Ted Kaptchuk has indicated that the 'Virtue' of the Wood Element is Humankindness. Kindness and generosity renew our life with meaning; tolerance helps us to forgive those who have made us angry.

Among the essentials of competent Shiatsu, the Wood Element may be equated with continuity. An easy continuity from one technique to the next is a sign of the smooth flow of the practitioner's Ki. Their treatment plan should unfold effortlessly, ensuring that diverse techniques are linked together smoothly.

Chapter 13

Fire: The Heart, Heart Protector, Small Intestines and Triple Heater

The ascending energy of Wood culminates in the expansion of Fire. Its upward surge towards 'Heaven' leads it to the mind (or Shen) of the Fire Element, to the Self. Growth leads to wholeness, which is symbolized by the image of Fire: Fire both radiates from a central point and embraces its periphery with light. It evokes the formless dance of consciousness, and shines forth as Divine Ruler of the bodymind.

Joy and love are the principle emotions ascribed to the Fire Element because they are the natural expressions of pure Being, the basic ground of awareness. Whereas the Will emerges from below and the Soul reaches upwards, the Mind occupies the central residence of the Heart. It is emotional in nature because all feelings, including those of the other Elements, pour through it.

The season of Fire is Summer, when the life processes of Nature reach a high point of activity, and the Yang energy of the Sun is at its peak.

THE FUNCTIONS OF THE HEART

Of the four Organs within the Fire Element, the Heart is the most important. Its two primary functions are to govern the Blood and blood vessels and to house the Mind.

Governs the Blood The Heart governs the Blood in a way that is similar to its function in Western Medicine: it acts as a pump which circulates blood around the body. However, Oriental Medicine also states that the Heart is the site for the final stage of Blood production. According to Oriental Medicine it is in the Heart where the transformation of Food-Ki into Blood takes place. The Heart and the Blood are closely interdependent: the Heart ensures the Blood's vitality through its proper circulation, and the Blood in turn nourishes the Heart and helps it to anchor the Mind. Together they help determine the constitutional strength of an individual.

When the Ki or Blood of the Heart are weak, the circulation may be sluggish and the extremities cold. The person will feel tired and unenthusiastic.

A central function of the Heart unique to Oriental Medicine is that it houses the Mind (or Shen). There are five main aspects to the Mind, those of: basic consciousness; mental activity (including the emotional); thinking; memory; and sleep. When the Heart is in good health and properly nourished by the Blood, consciousness is clear and the thinking process normal. There will be a well-balanced emotional life, a strong memory and restful sleep. Because they nourish the Heart both the Blood and the Yin help to anchor the Mind and thus keep it calm and peaceful. A Mind which is harmonious is said to be discerned in eyes through which its brilliant sparkle shines.

Houses the Mind

When the Heart is undernourished by the Blood and Yin, the Mind becomes 'ungrounded' and hyperactive. Feelings in general are intensified, and excessive 'Joy' manifests in the form of nervousness and excitement. The person will feel 'on edge', and will be more vulnerable to fright and shock, as their centre of consciousness will be less stable. A Mind which is seriously disturbed may result in behaviour which would be classified as 'manic' by Western Medicine.

An obviously milder and more common condition frequently involving the Fire Element is anxiety; a feeling of unease which includes a degree of both worry (Earth) and apprehension (Water). Again, the Mind cannot settle and occupy its residence within the Heart. Such distress may be compounded by a lack of Joy.

As part of its function of ruling the Blood, the Heart also controls the blood vessels. A healthy Heart will mean strong blood vessels and a clear, regular pulse.

Controls the Blood Vessels

That the Heart manifests in the complexion demonstrates the link between a healthy circulation and a lustrous, rosy complexion.

Manifests in the Complexion

The tongue is considered to be an extension of the Heart, and reflects in its shape and colour the condition of the Heart. Although the tongue shows the condition of all the Organs, it has particular bearing on that of the Heart. Heat in the Heart will often cause red, painful tongue ulcers as well as a bitter taste. The Heart also controls speech, and disharmonies occasionally lead to speech impediments such as stuttering. Heart problems may also mean that a person will talk incessantly or laugh without reason.

The Heart Opens Into the Tongue

Because of the close relationship between the Blood and Body Fluids,

Controls Sweat

the Heart controls sweat. When the Heart-Ki is weak there may be spontaneous sweating; a lack of Heart-Yin often leads to sweating at night.

THE FUNCTIONS OF THE HEART PROTECTOR

Although the Heart Protector (or Pericardium) is paired with the Triple Heater, it is in reality closely related to the Heart. Forming the outer covering of the Heart, it protects it against external pathogenic invasion (mainly Heat). The Heart Protector will bear the brunt of any such attack in order to shield the Mind from danger. When such situations do occur they involve External Heat causing high fever and delirium.

The Heart Protector also aids the Heart in functions of governing the Blood and housing the Mind. The Tsubos of the Heart Protector Channel are as important as those of the Heart, and can be used to treat the same conditions. Psychologically, the condition of the Heart is indicative of one's relationship with one's Self, whereas that of the Heart Protector reflects the way we relate to others. Treatment of the Heart Protector Channel is often appropriate for people experiencing distress in relationships.

THE FUNCTIONS OF THE SMALL INTESTINES

The function of the Small Intestines is to separate pure from impure food and fluids. It receives food and drink which has been 'rotted and ripened' by the Stomach, and continues the process of transformation by separating the 'clean' part for distribution by the Spleen. The 'dirty' part is transported to the Large Intestines for its excretion in the form of stools, and to the Bladder to be eliminated as urine. The Small Intestines' function of discrimination extends to the mental sphere in the form of decision-making. In this way it has an influence on the clarity of the Mind's thought processes.

Disharmonies of the Small Intestines are closely related to those of the Spleen, as both organs are central to the transformation of nourishment.

THE FUNCTIONS OF THE TRIPLE HEATER

The Triple Heater is the only 'Organ' which does not possess a precise physical form in the same way as the other twelve Officials. It comprises Three 'Heaters' (or 'Burners'): the Upper Heater occupies the thorax; the Middle Heater the space between the diaphragm and the navel; and the Lower Heater the area below the navel.

Each Heater produces Body Fluids with a different form and function: the Upper Heater can be compared to a 'mist', distributing fluids throughout the body as a 'vapour'; the Middle Heater is likened to a 'bubbling cauldron', the site of digestion and the transportation of nutrients; and the Lower Heater is like a 'drainage ditch', from which fluids are separated and excreted. It is the work of the Triple Heater as an Organ to ensure the free passage of Body Fluids between these three regions, and to help regulate their distinctive functions. Thus, according to 'The Yellow Emperor's Classic': 'The Triple Heater is the Official in charge of irrigation and the control of the water passages.'

The breadth of the Triple Heater's function is due to its intimate connection with the Gate of Vitality (*Ming Men*), located between the Kidneys at the Tsubo Governor Vessel-4. It is the Triple Heater which directs the Original Ki (the Ki derived from the Essence) from the Gate of Vitality to every Organ and Channel of the body. The Triple Heater thereby helps to warm the Organs, sustain the Heart and energize the brain – all through distributing the Original Ki generated in the Hara. By extending the Original Ki to the body's periphery, the Triple Heater furthermore contributes to the strength of the Defensive Ki, thus helping to protect the body.

A secondary aspect of its warming and protecting function is its role in supporting the fascia which insulate the organs, i.e. the pleura, peritoneum and diaphragm.

The Triple Heater Channel should always be treated whenever there is a lack of strength in the Hara. It can be used to both support the Original Ki and move Ki in the entire body. This latter function makes it useful whenever stagnant Ki accumulates, especially in the Liver, Stomach and Large Intestines. The Triple Heater Channel may be treated in cases of chronic debility, coldness, constipation, parietal headache and ear infection.

SHIATSU TREATMENT OF THE HEART AND HEART PROTECTOR

The Heart and Heart Protector are of great importance in Shiatsu for the role they can play in the treatment of mental and emotional problems. A general sign of Heart distress is seen in the patient who is anxious and complains of palpitations. The exact nature of the condition is revealed by other signs and symptoms.

Deficiency of Heart-Ki manifests as tiredness, pallor, sweating, palpitations and shortness of breath on exertion. There may well be anxiety and sadness. The pulse will be Empty and the tongue pale.

Treatment of Heart-Ki Deficiency

Administer tonifying Shiatsu to the Channel you find most Kyo. This will commonly be the Heart or Heart Protector, Kidney or Spleen. However don't assume this. Always check the Channels through Hara and Channel diagnosis (see chapter 18).

The main Tsubos to tonify Heart-Ki are Heart-5, Pericardium-6, Bladder-15 (the Heart Yu Point), and Directing Vessel-17 (which strengthens the Ki of the chest). Directing Vessel-6 should be tonified to raise the Ki of the whole body.

Treatment of Heart-Blood Deficiency

Deficiency of Blood affecting the Heart presents itself with symptoms which include palpitations, dizziness and a dull, pale complexion. The Blood's failure in helping the Heart to house the Mind leads to a poor memory, insomnia, and troubled, dream-filled sleep. It also means that the patient is likely to be anxious and easily startled. They will sometimes feel unable to cope with their responsibilities. The pulse will be Thready or Choppy; the tongue will be dry and a dull pale colour.

As usual, tonify the *most* Kyo Channel as diagnosed by reading the body, rather than automatically assume it will be the Heart or Heart Protector Channel.

The Tsubo Heart-7 should be tonified as it nourishes the Blood and calms the Mind. Heart-Blood may also be strengthened through the treatment of Directing Vessel-15, excellent for allaying deep anxiety. Important Tsubos for the tonification of Blood in general include Bladder-17 (Yu Point of the Blood), Bladder-20 (Yu Point of the Spleen) and Directing Vessel-4.

Treatment of Heart-Yin Deficiency

This pattern presents itself as an array of symptoms which combine those of deficient Yin with those of a troubled Heart. The condition is similar to that of deficient Heart-Blood, as in both cases the Mind becomes agitated, deprived of its 'home'.

Symptoms of Heart-Yin deficiency include palpitations, anxiety and restlessness, There will again be a failing memory, insomnia and sleep which is disturbed by dreams. However, there will also be the typical Yin deficient signs of feeling hot or slightly feverish, of sweating at night, and of thirst and a dry mouth. Also, the patient may have red cheeks, and hot hands and feet.

In this condition, the Heart and Heart Protector Channels should be Kyo and in need of tonification. (If they are Jitsu, the condition is likely to be a Full one such as Heart-Fire.) Heart-Yin Deficiency also requires the tonification of Kidney-Yin, upon which it relies for nourishment.

Heart-6 is the main Tsubo along the Heart Channel to tonify the Heart-Yin. Directing Vessel-15 will strengthen the Heart and dispel anxiety and restlessness. Spleen-6 and Kidney-6 are important to tonify the Yin in general, as well as to calm the Mind. Finally, Directing Vessel-4 anchors the Mind through nourishing the Yin and Blood.

So far we have looked at Deficient patterns of Heart disharmony, all of which require tonifying Shiatsu treatment. If, however, symptoms involving the Heart are found on a person whose Heart Channel is clearly Jitsu, their condition is likely to be Full in nature. There could be Fire, excessive Phlegm or Stagnation of Blood in the Heart. Such problems are often more acute than those of an Empty nature, and should be approached with caution, calling for a gently dispersing style of treatment.

Treatment of Full Heart Conditions

Heart-Fire is distinguished by feelings of heat throughout the day and night, by a red face, a bitter taste in the mouth, tongue ulcers and blood in the urine. There is usually a significant degree of mental agitation, occasionally combined with excessively extrovert or manic behaviour. Insomnia is also common. The pulse will be Rapid and Full; the tongue will be red (especially at the tip) and have a yellow coating. The Heart and Heart Protector Channels will almost certainly be Jitsu in condition. Dispersal of the Tsubos Heart-8 and -9 are called for, as they both clear Heart-Fire.

Heart-Fire Blazing

When Phlegm 'mists the orifices' of the Heart, there is often severe mental disturbance and confusion, as the Mind becomes seriously clouded and loses touch with reality. The pulse will be Rapid, Full and Slippery and the tongue red with a thick yellow coating. The Heart and Heart Protector Channels will most likely be Jitsu in condition. Check the Spleen Channel for a Kyo condition, as Spleen deficiency will contribute to the production of Phlegm. However, if another Channel is more Kyo, tonify that one instead. Heart Protector-5 is the main Tsubo to clear Phlegm from the Heart and 'open the orifices', and should naturally be dispersed.

Phlegm in the Heart

Stagnant Heart-Blood is an advanced pathological condition of the Heart involving chest pain which often radiates down the left arm. The chest feels stuffy or constricted and the nails, lips and tongue may be purple or blue. The Heart, Heart Protector, Liver and Gall Bladder Channels, if found to be Jitsu in condition, should be dispersed to move Blood in the chest. The main Tsubos for stagnation of Heart-Blood are Heart Protector-6 and Conception Vessel-17, both of which strengthen the Heart and promote the flow of Blood.

Stagnation of Heart-Blood

THE SPIRIT OF FIRE

The Heart is the 'Supreme Governor' of the bodymind, and was equated by the ancient Chinese with the role of Emperor. Its imperial position among the twelve main Organs is directly related to its function of housing the Shen. The Shen encompasses every aspect of human consciousness, uniting each emotional, mental and spiritual activity into a single whole. All the five Elements contribute to the creation of Selfhood: Water gives it drive; Wood, vision; Earth allows it form; and Metal, relationship. But it is Fire which *represents* this Selfhood and gives it its uniqueness and cohesion. 'The Shen are that by which a given being is unlike another; that which makes an individual an individual and more than merely a person.'[1]

The Fire Element presides over the bodymind as its 'Divine Ruler', granting it the capacity for enjoyment and love. It is Fire's responsibility to reconcile the instinctive with the rational, the emotional with the spiritual, and to maintain their delicate equilibrium. The power to harmonize these often conflicting activities requires a sense of perfection. This sense is linked to the 'Virtue' of the Fire Element, which, according to Ted Kaptchuk, is Propriety: a fine intuition for what is fit and proper.

To help restore equilibrium to the unsettled Shen of a recipient calls for Shiatsu which is truly effortless and non-judgemental. This requires an empty mind – one of the essentials of competent Shiatsu. An empty mind will allow us to work from the Heart. At one with the Hara, we are able to convey and awaken Ki; at one with the Heart, we can centre and harmonize the Shen.

NOTES

1. Claude Larre, Jean Schatz and Elisabeth Rochat de la Vallee, *Survey of Traditional Chinese Medicine*, translated by Sarah Elizabeth Stang (Institut Ricci, Paris, and Traditional Acupuncture Institute, 1986), p.192.

Chapter 14

Earth: The Spleen and Stomach

The Earth Element takes the basic consciousness of Fire and gives it form. It does this through the creation of concrete thought, and putting ideas into action. Water imbues life with impetus, Wood harnesses it; Fire crowns life with self-awareness and now Earth must give it focus. Each Element nourishes the next. The self-orientation of Fire compensates for the goal-orientation of Wood; similarly, Earth's concern with the real modifies Fire's emphasis on the ideal. The Earth Element thus allows the Mind a vehicle through which it can explore and express itself on a practical level.

The nature of the Earth Element is to consolidate and maintain. Among the Five Elements it is one which occupies the Centre, the position from which it can most effectively bind together and sustain the other four. In order to nurture the bodymind it must be capable of absorption. However, crucial to absorption is the power to take that which is 'other' and make it one's own. This is the process central to Earth: that of transformation.

Earth's transformative function is apparent on two main levels: that of the digestion of food and its final conversion into Blood; and that of the process of mental cognition and Thought (Yi). Earth absorbs the sensations and perceptions of the bodymind, breaks them down like the soil, and makes them part of the Mind. This gives credence to the sympathetic nature of Earth, as does its urge to nurture.

Only transformation which is efficient yields productive results. Overthinking, the 'emotion' of Earth, often means remaining stuck in repetitive cycles of thought. This prevents energy from descending towards the earth, towards the realm of action. When Thought cannot reach conclusions and transform into reality then worry and obsessiveness ensue. Giving sympathy to someone soothes and settles their thoughts and helps them find understanding.

The nurturing aspect of Earth is an important one and is clearly reflected in the functions of its associated Organs, the Stomach and Spleen. The Stomach is the ultimate source of the body's nourishment and the Spleen the origin of the Blood. Together they play the role of Mother Earth, providing the body with sustenance.

THE FUNCTIONS OF THE SPLEEN

The Spleen is the primary Zang Organ of the Earth Element, and includes the pancreas as part of its functional unit.

Governs Transformation and Transportation

The first function of the Spleen is the transformation of ingested food and drink into Food-Ki, and the transportation of nutrients to the other bodily viscera. Food-Ki provides the raw material for the manufacture of Ki and Blood. It is derived from the 'pure essence' of food and is directed upwards by the Spleen to the Lungs and Heart. It is in the chest that Food-Ki combines with the 'Ki of clean air' to form Gathering Ki, and in the Heart that it is converted into Blood.

The Spleen is the main Organ of digestion due to its central role of transformation and transportation, and is the source of bodily Ki and Blood. Its importance is highlighted by the fact that it is the foundation of 'Post-Heaven Essence' (see p.127). The Spleen is also responsible for the transformation, separation and transportation of fluids. The 'clear' Body Fluids go to the Lungs for dispersal around the body and the 'dirty' part enters the intestines for further refinement.

A healthy Spleen ensures that digestion and absorption are efficient and normal, that there is a good appetite, and that bowel movements are regular. If this process is disrupted, digestion will be upset and the appetite poor. There will be abdominal swelling, loose stools and the accumulation of excessive Body Fluids in the form of Dampness, Phlegm or oedema.

Controls the Blood

The Spleen is not only responsible for the origin of Blood through the transformation of food, but 'controls' the Blood by keeping it in the blood vessels. A breakdown of this function may lead to such problems as haemorrhage or excessive menstrual bleeding.

Controls the Muscles and the Four Limbs

Because the Spleen is the basis of nourishment and its transportation around the body, it plays a major role in ensuring muscular strength, and thus 'controls' the muscles and the four limbs.

Opens into the Mouth and Manifests in the Lips

The action of chewing is the first stage in the transformation of food, and for this reason is closely connected to the Spleen. The Spleen, therefore, opens into the mouth and manifests in the lips. The Spleen produces the sense of taste as well as a feeling of appetite. Spleen dysfunction will manifest in either dry, cracked lips, indicating the presence of Heat, or pale lips, showing that Spleen-Ki is weak.

In addition to raising Food-Ki to the chest, the Spleen has the function of controlling the raising of Ki in a general sense. It 'lifts' the internal organs and so holds them in their proper place. Failure of this function leads to prolapse or herniation.

Controls the Raising of Ki

Finally, the Spleen houses 'Thought', dominating the processes of thinking, analysing, concentrating and studying. In health, the Spleen ensures strong powers of reasoning and memory. When there is a deficiency of Spleen-Ki, the thought process will be unclear and the concentration cloudy. Such a person may have to expend a lot of mental energy in finding solutions, resulting in Overthinking and a further depletion of Spleen-Ki.

Houses Thought (Yi)

THE FUNCTIONS OF THE STOMACH

The Stomach is perhaps the most important Yang Organ, forming, in conjunction with the Spleen, the 'Root of Post-Heaven Ki'. Pre-Heaven Ki, assimilated before birth by the Kidneys, is the source of our consitutional strength, whereas Post-Heaven Ki is formed after birth by the Stomach and Spleen from food and drink. Both the Earth Organs have a major influence on the quality of Ki and Blood.

The primary function of the Stomach is to control the 'rotting and ripening' of food. Through a process akin to fermentation, food is prepared by the Stomach for its refinement by the Spleen and its separation by the Small Intestines. Representing the first stage in the digestive process, it forms the very basis of bodily nourishment.

Controls the Rotting and Ripening of Food

Along with the Spleen, the Stomach also controls the transportation of food essences to the entire body, particularly the muscles and limbs. If the Stomach-Ki is weak, the legs and arms will feel heavy and the person will easily tire.

Controls the Transportation of Food Essences

The Stomach is said to control the descending of Ki by virtue of its action in sending down food to the Small Intestines. Whereas Spleen-Ki ascends and controls the raising of Ki, Stomach-Ki should descend. Failure of this Stomach function, often because of its disruption by Liver-Ki Stagnation, will lead to bloating, belching, gastric reflux, hiccup and vomiting – all signs of Stomach-Ki 'rebelling' upward.

Controls the Descending of Ki

SHIATSU TREATMENT OF THE SPLEEN AND STOMACH

Spleen and Stomach Deficiency

A deficiency of Spleen-Ki produces a host of symptoms centring around weakness in the digestive processes and a resulting lack of available energy. Besides a dragging feeling of tiredness and weakness in the limbs, there is abdominal swelling, a lack of appetite, loose stools and a pale complexion. Spleen-Ki deficiency produces an Empty pulse and a tongue which may be pale and swollen.

Dampness and Phlegm may also accumulate due to an impaired transformation function. This is evident in fluid retention, feelings of heaviness and respiratory congestion. Dampness and Phlegm produce a Slippery pulse and tongue with a thick and sticky coating. In the case of Spleen-Yang deficiency, we can add to these symptoms feelings of cold, especially in the limbs. The pulse will be Deep and Weak and the tongue pale, swollen and wet.

A deficiency of Stomach-Ki will manifest the same symptoms, but with a greater emphasis on discomfort in the epigastric area. The pulse will be Empty and the tongue pale. When the Spleen and Stomach are deficient, their Channels will usually be Kyo in condition. The diagnostic area for the Spleen on the Hara (around the navel) will often be swollen or puffy and feel Empty to the touch.

The treatment of these deficient Spleen and Stomach patterns may be approached in basically the same way. In both cases tonify the Spleen and Stomach Channels, including the Tsubos Spleen-6 and Stomach-36. Treat the Tsubos Directing Vessel-12 (Bo point for the Stomach and Middle Heater) and Bladder-20 and -21 (Spleen and Stomach Yu Points). All these Tsubos have a strong tonifying action, especially when there are signs of Cold.

Excessive Dampness, especially when it has invaded the Spleen itself, may produce a Jitsu condition in the Spleen and Stomach Channels. Dispersing the Spleen and Stomach Channels as well as the Tsubo Stomach-40 will help clear Dampness and Phlegm.

The Spleen Channel is often Kyo in condition when there is Blood deficiency, evident in signs of dizziness, tiredness, dry skin, cracked nails and impaired vision. It is important in this case to tonify both the Spleen and Stomach Channels and so strengthen the digestion. It may also be necessary to tonify the Liver and Heart Channels, because these Organs are easily affected by Blood deficiency.

Retention of Food in the Stomach

When the Stomach-Ki stagnates, often due to Liver-Ki stagnation, a 'stuck' condition manifests and causes a sensation of abdominal fullness and bloating. Food is not properly digested and is 'retained' in the Stomach, leading to appetite loss, nausea and signs of Stomach-Ki 'rebelling' upwards, i.e. belching, acid regurgitation and vomiting. The pulse will be Full and Slippery or Wiry; the tongue will have a thick coating.

The Stomach Channel is usually Jitsu in this condition. Tsubos which relieve the Retention of Food and encourage Stomach-Ki to descend include Stomach-21 and Stomach-44.

Stomach-Yin Deficiency

The Stomach is said to be the origin of fluids in the body, and unlike the Spleen, can become deficient in Yin. This will produce symptoms of dryness, including a dry mouth and throat, thirst, and dry stools which lead to constipation. These problems will be coupled with epigastric pain and appetite loss. The pulse will be Floating, and the tongue red and possibly peeled or cracked in the centre.

The Stomach Channel is very likely to be Kyo in condition. Check the Kidney Channel also, as the Kidneys will be involved in any Yin-deficient pattern. Specific Tsubos to tonify are Stomach-36, Spleen-6 and Directing Vessel-12.

Phlegm-Fire in the Stomach

When Phlegm and Fire build up in the Stomach due to poor dietary habits, a Full condition ensues. Stomach Phlegm-Fire is characterized by feelings of burning and pain in the Stomach area, by constant hunger, bleeding gums, constipation, nausea and bad breath. There is often a strong desire to drink cold liquids in order to quell the Fire. Mentally, insomnia and worry are common. The more that Phlegm is involved, the greater the sense of congestion and disorientation. The pulse will be Rapid and Full due to Heat and possibly Slippery due to Phlegm. The tongue will be red with a thick, yellow coating.

Check the Stomach Channel: it is likely to be Jitsu and in need of dispersal. Disperse the Tsubos Stomach-21 and Stomach-44, both of which clear Heat from the Stomach. Disperse Stomach-40 to clear Phlegm.

THE SPIRIT OF EARTH

As thinking precedes physical action, it seems appropriate that Thought should be associated with the Earth Element. Thought is the first stage in the process of actualization, i.e. bringing ideas into reality. The higher purpose of Thought, and the 'Virtue' of the Earth Element,[3] is to explore the creative possibilities of the Mind.

Creativity is an alchemical process; taking the base metals of the Mind and converting them into the gold of art and philosophy. True art requires a sense of proportion and harmony – something which Thought derives from the Propriety of the Shen. At the same time, creativity releases us from the strictures of Propriety, and encourages us to explore the realm of the possible.

Creativity in Shiatsu is akin to fluency, an essential aspect of competent treatment. Fluency is the ability to draw on a wide variety of techniques in direct response to the recipient's needs. All techniques, however, should be based on the stable ground of support, another keynote of Earth.

Chapter 15

Metal: The Lungs and Large Intestines

Once the Earth Element has established consciousness on a physical plane it is left to Metal to complete the making of the Self by lending it boundary. Paradoxically, having a surface – a skin – allows us to interact with others and the environment; it provides us with a transmission point across which we can 'take in' and 'let go'.

The Metal Element is symbolic of our constant partaking of life, and is seen at work in the breath. It says, 'We are what passes through us,' and defines the Self according to its interaction with the external world. The more that we can 'open up' to our environment and at the same time relinquish the things of the past, the more vital and alive we are. This vitality is a manifestation of the Corporeal Soul or P'o, closely linked to the Lungs and the Metal Element in general.

Whereas the Ethereal Soul is future-orientated, the bodily or Corporeal Soul is concerned only with the present. The Corporeal Soul may be compared to the vibrant, ever-fresh world of young children, ceaselessly immersed in the exploration of the things around them.

Thus, when we lose someone or something dear to us, it is this very capacity – to be always in the moment – which loses hold. Our minds centre for a while on the past, as we go through a special process called Grief. It is only through grieving that we can learn a deeper acceptance of life and death, and therefore regain the present.

If, however, we never fully grieve, we are likely to remain 'stuck' in an acute awareness of what we have lost, and become melancholic and remorseful. The boundary between us and present reality will grow, and others will feel that we are 'out of reach' in some way. Such a person becomes dominated by the Metal Element because they cannot learn the process which is central to it: that of accepting and 'letting go'.

THE FUNCTIONS OF THE LUNGS

The functions of the Lungs are directly related to the process of respiration, and indirectly to the Heart and circulation.

Govern Ki and Respiration

When the Lungs inhale air they are extracting 'pure Ki' from their environment. Exhalation is a way of discharging 'dirty Ki'. Respiration thus ensures the continual renewal and freshness of bodily Ki.

The Lungs also dominate the formation of Ki in the chest. Food-Ki, made from refined food and drink, is directed by the Spleen up to the chest, where it combines with the 'pure Ki' of air to form Gathering Ki or 'Ki of the chest'. Gathering Ki forms the basis of Nutritive and Defensive Ki, and lends force to Lung and Heart function. A deficiency of Lung-Ki will directly affect the Ki of the whole body.

Control the Channels and Blood Vessels

Because the Lungs govern the Ki and Ki propels the Heart and circulation, the Lungs are said to control both the Channels and blood vessels. The Lungs are the most important Organ in the formation of Nutritive Ki, the Ki which flows not only in the Channels, but in the blood vessels as well. The circulation of Ki and Blood are closely connected, as the Blood relies on the Ki for its propulsion around the body. They are both greatly influenced by the strength of the Lung-Ki.

Control Dispersing and Descending

This important Lung function is associated with the Lungs' control of the Ki. The Lungs control the dispersing of both Defensive Ki and Body Fluids around the periphery of the body – to the space between the muscles and skin. When the Defensive Ki is spread evenly under the body surface it fulfils the role of protecting the body from pathogenic factors such as Cold and Dampness. It also warms the skin and muscles. Impairment of this function will cause a weakening of Defensive Ki and pave the way for invasion of the body by pathogenic factors, causing ailments such as colds and influenza.

The dispersal of Body Fluids by the Lungs ensures that sufficient moisture reaches the skin and muscles. The Body Fluids are distributed in the form of a 'fine mist'. (This is the form in which they appear in the region of the Upper Heater.) The Lungs also regulate the opening and closing of the pores on the skin surface. They ensure that perspiration is normal, i.e. neither excessive or deficient.

The Lungs have an important descending function. As they are the uppermost Organ of the body, it is important that their energy descends in order for Ki to 'communicate' with the rest of the body. The Lungs therefore have an important relationship with the Kidneys. The Lungs send Ki downwards and the Kidneys 'grasp' it. The Lungs also descend and provide Ki for the functioning of the Bladder and Large Intestines. This descending function further pertains to the downward movement of Body Fluids by the Lungs.

Impairment of the Lung's descending function will lead to Ki and body fluids becoming 'stuck' in the thorax, causing coughing and a congested feeling in the chest.

As we have seen, the Lungs play an important role in the distribution of Body Fluids. First, they disperse the Body Fluids throughout the periphery of the body, and secondly, they descend the Body Fluids to the Kidneys and Bladder. For this reason, they are considered to regulate the water passages. Failure of the Lungs to adequately disperse and descend Body Fluids often leads to slight water retention in the face.

Regulate the Water Passages

Because the Lungs disperse the Ki and ensure that the body surface receives adequate nourishment and moisture, the Lungs are said to control the skin and hair. If the Body Fluids are properly dispersed by the Lungs, the skin will be lustrous and the hair shiny. If not, the skin will become dry and body hair brittle and withered.

Control the Skin and Hair

The Lungs open into the nose, the gateway of the breath. When the Lungs are invaded by an external pathogenic factor, the nose easily becomes blocked and there is frequent sneezing. Sneezing is a sign that the descending of Lung-Ki is being obstructed.

Open into the Nose

Finally, the Lungs house the Corporeal Soul. We have already looked at the nature of the Corporeal Soul and the way in which it is affected by Grief. Feelings of sadness will also constrict the Corporeal Soul. This will in turn inhibit breathing and therefore blunt vitality. Otherwise, the Corporeal Soul is naturally optimistic and open to new experiences.

House the Corporeal Soul

THE FUNCTIONS OF THE LARGE INTESTINES

The functions of the Large Intestines are very simple: it receives food and drink from the Small Intestines, absorbs the remaining 'clean' fluids, and excretes the 'dirty' portion of food in the form of stools.

If the Lungs fail in their descending function, the Large Intestines may not receive sufficient Ki to ensure defecation. This will give rise to constipation, which is common with elderly people in whom Lung-Ki is often deficient.

Western naturopathic medicine recognizes that a loss of its appropriate bacterial colonization in the Large Intestines undermines health and weakens the immune system. Oriental Medicine also makes a connection between a healthy Large Intestine and the strength of the Defensive (Wei) Ki.

SHIATSU TREATMENT OF THE LUNGS

Weakness of Lung-Ki can develop as a result of spending long hours

Lung-Ki Deficiency

stooped over a desk. It can also come about through repeated chest infections which have not been properly treated, allowing External Wind to penetrate deeper into the Lungs.

Deficiency of Lung-Ki is apparent from a lack of vitality, shortness of breath, a weak voice, spontaneous sweating and possibly cough. The face will have a bright, white colour. Such a condition will also lead to a deficiency of Defensive Ki, resulting in the frequent occurrence of respiratory infections. The pulse will be Empty and the tongue pale.

Check for a Kyo condition of the Lung Channel, and possibly the Heart Channel as well. Administer tonifying Shiatsu treatment if the Kyo condition is confirmed, concentrating on the Tsubos Lung-9, Lung-7 and Bladder-13, all of which tonify Lung-Ki.

Lung-Yin Deficiency   When the Yin of the Lungs are deficient, one sees symptoms of Yin-deficiency (feelings of heat, a dry mouth and throat, thirst, insomnia, night sweats and so on) together with symptoms which indicate a Lung problem. These include a dry cough with very little mucus, sputum tinged with blood, and a hoarse voice. The pulse will be Floating; the tongue will be red, dry and possibly peeled or cracked in the Lung area.

It is again necessary to check whether the Lung Channel is Kyo in condition, together with that of the Kidneys, as the Kidneys are the source of Yin in the body. Shiatsu treatment should again be tonifying in nature, and include the Tsubos Lung-9, and Bladder-43, both of which tonify Lung-Yin. Kidney-Yin may be strengthened through the tonification of the Tsubo Kidney-6.

Invasion of the Lungs by Wind   The Lungs are considered to be the most exterior Organ of the body and have a strong influence on the Defensive Ki. When External pathogenic Wind invades the Defensive level of the body, the resulting struggle between the invading Wind and the Defensive Ki leads to fever. The Lungs' dispersing and descending function becomes impaired and causes the usual symptoms of a cold: cough, sneezing and blocked sinuses and so on. One feels tired and achy. Symptoms involving External Wind can be classified according to Cold and Hot types.

Wind-Cold is in evidence when the body feels chilled and mildly feverish, when nasal mucus is clear and watery, the throat is itchy, and there is an absence of thirst and sweating. Headaches arising from Wind-Cold are centred on the back of the head. The tongue is covered by a thin, white coating.

Wind-Heat is characterized by a stronger fever, nasal mucus which is yellow, and a sore, often swollen throat. There is usually thirst and sweating. Headaches arising from Wind-Heat are often more severe, and are not limited to the occiput. The tongue is covered by a thin, yellow coating.

Those with fever generally have an aversion to being touched. However, if you find the Lung, Large Intestine or Triple Heater to be Jitsu, you *may* be able to apply careful sedation techniques to release the

External Wind. Shiatsu Treatment should be concentrated around the upper back and chest area. The Tsubo Bladder-12 disperses External Wind of both the Cold and Hot type. Disperse Lung-7 in the case of Wind-Cold; Large Intestine-4 and Triple Heater-5 in the case of Wind-Heat. Dispersal of the Tsubo Gall Bladder-20 will relieve headaches due to the invasion of External Wind.

Phlegm Obstructing the Lungs

In the Creation Cycle of the Five Elements the Earth Element is mother to Metal. It is therefore common for excessive Dampness produced by the Spleen to collect in the Lungs. This tends to occur in people who eat a high proportion of Damp-forming foods such as dairy products, sugar and raw food.

The Phlegm that accumulates obstructs breathing and causes coughing and the expectoration of profuse amounts of whitish sputum. The chest feels congested, there is shortness of breath and the complexion is white and pasty. The pulse is Slippery and the tongue has a thick, white coating.

Phlegm which is retained in the Lungs for long periods of time tends to become Phlegm-Heat. This becomes apparent in the production of sputum which is thick and yellow or green. The resulting cough has a barking quality, and there is again shortness of breath.

Check the Lung and Spleen Channels for either a Jitsu or Kyo condition. Treat the Channels accordingly, concentrating on the chest, Kyo, despite the fact that the presence of Phlegm indicates a Full condition. Treat the Channels accordingly concentrating on the chest, upper back and upper Hara. Specific Tsubos should include Lung-5 (for expelling Phlegm and Heat from the Lungs), Lung-7 (stimulating Lung descending function and stopping cough), Stomach-40 (excellent for clearing Phlegm) and Bladder-13 and -20 (Lung and Spleen Yu Points).

Symptomatic relief of obstruction by Phlegm can also be achieved by Shiatsu applied directly to the rib cage (see p.112).

SHIATSU TREATMENT OF THE LARGE INTESTINES

Problems which are common to the Large Intestines, such as constipation and diarrhoea, frequently find their root in other Organs, particularly the Liver and Spleen. Like the Lungs, the Large Intestines can also be invaded by external pathogenic factors such as Heat and Cold.

Damp-Heat in the Large Intestines

This problem arises from eating too many greasy foods, allowing Dampness to build-up in the Large Intestines. Again, Dampness may turn to Damp-Heat over a certain period of time. The problem is characterized by diarrhoea, burning in the anus, strong-smelling stools, abdominal pain, fever, thirst and a feeling of heaviness.

Check the Large Intestine, Spleen and Stomach Channels for either a Jitsu or Kyo condition. As the problem is Full in nature, they are more likely to be Jitsu in condition. Treat them accordingly, giving particular attention to treatment of the Hara. Specific Tsubos should include Stomach-25 (Bo Point of the Large Intestine; stops diarrhoea), Spleen-6 and -9 (clear Dampness from the Lower Heater) and Large Intestine-11 (clears Heat from the bowels).

Cold Invading the Large Intestines

This problem arises when the Large Intestines are invaded by External Cold. It occurs when a person has been exposed to cold weather without sufficient clothing to keep the Hara warm. Invasion of Cold is characterized by acute abdominal pain, diarrhoea and feelings of cold, especially in the abdomen.

Like most Full conditions, some sedation of Jitsu may be required before Kyo can be found and tonified. Also, try treating the Hara directly. Concentrate treatment on these Channels and on the Hara. Disperse the Tsubos Stomach-25 (Bo Point of the Large Intestines) and Stomach-36 (excellent for expelling Cold).

THE SPIRIT OF METAL

The Metal Element reflects both the capacity to be involved and responsive as well as that of being detached and separate. Its dual nature is like the breath: expanding and contracting, receiving and releasing. It teaches us to partake of life, but without trying to 'hold on to it'. It diminishes our sense of 'I' and, according to Ted Kaptchuk, teaches us the Virtue of Reverence.

Learning reverence and respect for the body are important aspects of healing. We so often seem to live to gratify our mind and senses, often at the expense of good health. Cultivating the body revitalizes mind and Spirit and fosters openness and optimism.

The essentials of competent Shiatsu which reflect the qualities of Metal are positive connection and steadiness of breath. Establishing a vital connection with the recipient allows for the maximum transmission of Ki, and enhances the feeling of communication inherent in Shiatsu. Steadiness of breath ensures an empty mind, both of which are prerequisites for a strong and open Hara.

Chapter 16

Kyo/Jitsu, Symptoms and Organ Function

Shizuto Masunaga presented a list of symptoms for the Kyo and Jitsu conditions of each major Channel. The symptoms he categorized were based on his own clinical observations and interpretation of Oriental Medicine and Western physiology. Although he firmly established Kyo/Jitsu methodology as a tool of diagnosis in its own right, the many different physical and psychological symptoms which he ascribed to it were not always clearly explained.

As a means of summarizing the functions and disharmonies of the Organs, we have taken many of the key physical and psychological symptoms listed by Masunaga, and explained them in a way that demonstrates their direct relationship to Organ function according to Oriental Medicine.

KYO/JITSU AND SYMPTOMS OF THE YIN ORGANS

Kidney Kyo

Symptom	Explanation
Chronic fatigue	Kidneys are the root of Yang
Excessive urination	Kidneys control Water
Poor circulation in the hips and Hara	Kidneys warm the Lower Heater
Lower back ache	Kidneys warm the Lower Heater; Kidney Marrow fills the spine
Weak sexual vitality	Kidney-Essence governs reproduction and harmonizes sexual function; Kidney-Yang mobilizes Essence
Brittle/soft bones	Kidney Marrow controls the bones

Symptoms	*Explanation*
Poor nails	Kidney Marrow helps make Blood
Thirst/dry mouth and throat	Kidney-Yin deficiency
Anxiety/restlessness/insomnia	Kidneys fail to anchor the Mind; Kidney-Yin deficiency
Lack of will/endurance	Kidneys fail to house the Will (*Zhi*)
Fear/apprehension	Fear is the emotion of the Water Element

Kidney Jitsu

Symptom	*Explanation*
Thirst/dark urine/blood in the urine	Kidney-Yin deficiency causing Heat in the Kidneys
Nosebleeds/fainting/heaviness in head/bitter taste in mouth	Kidney-Yin deficiency causing rising Excess Yang
Inflamed throat	Kidney-Yin deficiency and Kidney-Heat leading to Lung-Heat
Ringing in the ears	Kidneys open into the ears; Kidney-Yin deficiency causing rising Yang
Back stiffness	Kidneys control the Lower Heater
Excessive sexual drive	Kidney-Yin deficiency
Impatience/restlessness/work-aholic	Kidney disharmony causing hyperactive Will (*Zhi*)

Liver Kyo

Symptom	*Explanation*
Fatigue/dizziness/dull pale complexion	Liver fails to store the Blood, causing Blood deficiency
Cracked nails	Liver-Blood manifests in the nails
Infertility	Liver-Blood important to nourish the Uterus
Weak eyes/'floaters' in the eyes	Liver-Blood fails to nourish the eyes

Symptoms	*Explanation*
Weak joints/stiff muscles	Liver controls the tendons ('sinews')
Irritability/depression	Depressed Liver Ki affects the emotions
Lack of determination/inconsistent	'Liver [in health] is a resolute Organ'

Liver Jitsu

Symptom	*Explanation*
Exhaustion due to excessive drive	'Liver is a resolute Organ'
Swollen epigastrium/poor digestion/flatulence	Liver Ki stagnation invades the Stomach
Headaches	Liver Ki stagnation/Liver-Yang rising
Chronic stiffness/tightness in Hara	Liver Ki stagnation affecting the sinews and muscles
Haemorrhoids/skin eruptions	Liver Heat transmitted to Blood
Inflammatory diseases of reproductive system	Liver Channel encircles genitals; Liver Fire
Excessive work and concentration/stubborn	'Liver is a resolute organ'
Frustrated/impatient/impulsive	Liver-Ki stagnation; Ki does not flow freely
Represses anger/explodes	Stagnation of the emotions

Heart Kyo

Symptom	*Explanation*
Poor circulation/fatigue	Heart governs Blood and circulation
Palpitations/angina pectoris	Deficiency of Heart-Yang, -Yin or -Blood
Stuttering/pulling sensation in the tongue	Heart opens into the tongue
Sweaty palms	Heart controls sweat
Weakness/tightness in upper Hara	Upper Hara is Heart diagnostic area
Nervous tension/over-sensitivity/shock	Heart houses the Mind (Shen)

Symptoms	*Explanation*
Anxiety/restlessness	Heart-Yin deficiency
Poor memory	Heart-Blood deficiency
Sadness/disappointment	Joy is the emotion of the Fire Element

Heart Jitsu

Symptom	*Explanation*
Palpitations/chest pain	Heart-Blood stagnation/Heart-Fire blazing
Poor circulation	Heart-Blood stagnation
Ulcers on the tongue	Heart opens into the tongue; Heart-Fire blazing
Heavy perspiration	Heart controls sweat
Stiffness/fullness in the upper Hara	Heart diagnostic area
Nervousness/restlessness/over-excitement	Heart houses the Mind (Shen); excessive 'Joy'
Hysteria/mania/excessive, inappropriate laughter	Full condition of the Heart; a Mind agitated by Heat or Fire

Heart Governor Kyo

Symptoms	*Explanation*
Palpitations/breathless on exertion/weak pulse	Deficient Ki of the Heart and Heart Governor
Poor circulation and cold limbs	Deficient Yang of Heart and Heart Governor
Anxiety/restlessness/insomnia	Deficient Yin of Heart and Heart Governor
Emotional over-sensitivity in relationships	Heart Governor influences close relating

Heart Governor Jitsu

Symptoms	*Explanation*
Constriction, stuffiness and heaviness in the chest	Blood stagnation of Heart and Heart Governor
Palpitations/tongue and mouth ulcers/insomnia/heat	Fire in the Heart and Heart Governor

Symptoms	*Explanation*
Over-emotional/impulsive/ agitated, particularly in regard to relationships	Excessive 'Joy' and excitement

Spleen Kyo

Symptom	*Explanation*
Poor digestion/emaciation/ appetite loss/lethargy	Spleen's transformation function impaired
Accumulation of catarrh and phlegm	Spleen's transformation function impaired
Heavy, tired limbs	Spleen controls the muscles and four limbs
Anaemia	Spleen is the origin of Blood
Lack of saliva/lack of taste	Spleen opens into the mouth/fails to raise fluids
Pale gums	Spleen opens into the mouth
Prolapse	Spleen's raising of Ki function fails
Sleepiness	Spleen fails to raise Ki/Spleen Dampness affects head
Overthinking/worry/poor concentration	Spleen is the residence of Thought (Yi)
Craves sympathy and understanding	Spleen requires nurturing/is the Organ of consideration

Spleen Jitsu

Symptom	*Explanation*
Appetite loss/gastric hyperacidity	Spleen's transformation function impaired: accumulation of Phlegm-Heat
Sticky feeling in mouth/mucus in the Lungs	Poor transformation leads to Phlegm-Damp
Obesity	Poor transformation leads to Dampness and oedema
Heaviness in the legs/stiffness in the arms/lack of strength	Spleen controls the muscles and four limbs
Overthinking/obsessiveness/un- clear thinking	Spleen is the residence of Thought (Yi)

Symptoms	*Explanation*
Excessive concern for others/self-pity	Spleen is the Organ of nurturing/excessive Thought becomes worry

Lung Kyo

Symptom	*Explanation*
Difficulty breathing/cough/bronchitis	Lungs govern respiration
Fatigue, especially in upper body	Lungs govern Ki
Frequent colds/influenza	Lungs govern dispersing and descending function/Defensive Ki
Heaviness in the head	Lungs control the Channels and blood vessels
Unenthusiastic, negative attitude	Lungs house Corporeal Soul (*P'o*) source of one's vital spirit
Grief/melancholy	Grief is the emotion of the Metal Element

Lung Jitsu

Symptom	*Explanation*
Nasal and chest congestion	Phlegm-Damp obstructing the Lungs
Coughing pain in the chest	Full condition of the Lungs
Bronchitis	Heat and Phlegm in the Lungs
Asthma	Impairment of the Lungs dispersing and descending function
Tight chest/muscles	Stagnation of Ki in the chest
Pulling sensation in thumb	Lung Channel obstruction
Grief/oppression	Grief is the emotion of the Metal Element
Detachment/defensiveness/pride	Inability to 'open up'
Selfishness/jealousy	Inability to 'let go'

KYO/JITSU AND SYMPTOMS OF THE YANG ORGANS

Bladder Kyo

Symptom	*Explanation*
Frequent, pale, copious urination	Bladder fails to properly transform fluids due to Kidney-Yang deficiency
Incontinence	Bladder fails to control fluids due to Kidney-Yang deficiency
Poor circulation in the Hara and legs/cold and achy lower back	Kidney Yang fails to warm Lower Heater/Bladder deficiency with Cold
Fear and apprehension	Fear is the emotion of the Water Element

Bladder Jitsu

Symptom	*Explanation*
Frequent, urgent urination/difficult urination	Dampness in the Bladder obstructs the flow of fluids
Turbid, milky urine	Dampness in the Bladder
Heaviness and cramping in lower Hara	Dampness and Cold in the Bladder
Burning urination/blood in the urine	Heat in the Bladder
Tightness in the back of the legs	Obstruction of Bladder Channel
Jealousy and suspicion	Fear/inability to 'let go'

Gall Bladder Kyo

Symptom	*Explanation*
Dizziness/poor vision	Part of Liver-Blood deficiency pattern
Poor digestion of fats	Impairment of Gall Bladder function of bile secretion
Weak, tired legs	Gall Bladder Channel has an important influence on the legs
Timidity and lack of initiative	Gall Bladder is the source of courage

Gall Bladder Jitsu

Symptom

Pain and swelling under rib
  cage/nausea/loss of appetite

Poor digestion of fats/yellow
  complexion

Bitter taste in the mouth/dark
  urine

Gallstones

Stiff muscles along sides of
  body

Impatient/hurried/driven/over-
  ambitious

Irritable/frustrated/angry

Explanation

Dampness in the Gall Bladder/
  Stagnation of Liver-Ki

Secretion of bile obstructed by
  Dampness

Heat/inflammation in the Gall
  Bladder

'Substantial' Phlegm obstructs
  the Gall Bladder

Obstruction of Gall Bladder
  Channel

Initiative and 'courage' in
  excess

Anger is the emotion of the
  Wood Element

Small Intestines Kyo

Symptom

Abdominal pain/desire for hot
  drinks

Borborygmi (gurgling in the
  abdomen)

Diarrhoea

Lack of strength in Hara/poor
  circulation in hips

Shoulder pain

Indecision/lack of mental
  clarity

Explanation

Cold in the Small Intestines
  obstructs Ki-flow in abdomen
  – caused by Spleen-Yang
  Deficiency

Characteristic of Small
  Intestines disharmony

Small Intestines and Spleen fail
  to transform food and drink
  due to Yang Deficiency

Deficiency of Small Intestines;
  poor Ki-flow in Lower Heater

Obstruction of Small Intestines
  Channel

Small Intestines separates the
  pure from the impure

Small Intestines Jitsu

Symptoms

Abdominal swelling/twisting
  pain in abdomen

Explanation

Stagnation of Ki in the Small
  Intestines, caused by Liver-Ki
  stagnation

Symptoms	Explanation
Borborygmi/flatulence/constipation	Ki Stagnation impairs transformation function of Small Intestines
Abdominal pain with signs of Heat/thirst/restlessness/dark, scanty urine	Heat in the Small Intestines
Deafness	Fire in the Small Intestine Channel
Stiffness and pain in the shoulders and neck	Obstruction of the Small Intestine Channel
Mental restlessness/obsessiveness/indecision	Small Intestine separates the pure from the impure/influences the Heart and hence the Mind

Triple Heater Kyo

Symptoms	Explanation
Feelings of cold	Triple Heater fails to distribute warmth from the Gate of Vitality
Susceptibility to colds and flu	Ki deficiency of the Upper Heater
Abdominal swelling/indigestion/loose stools	Impairment of function of the Middle Heater
Oedema, swelling and Cold in the lower abdomen	Impairment of function of the Lower Heater
Socially unconfident/recluse	Exterior relationship to Heart Governor, influencing social communication
Unadventurous/timid	Lack of 'Joy'

Triple Heater Jitsu

Symptoms	Explanation
Earache/lateral headache/swollen cheeks/sore throat	External Wind invades the Triple Heater Channel
Indigestion/abdominal pain and heaviness	Stagnant Ki and Retention of Food in the Middle Heater
Constipation/fullness and tightness in the Hara	Stagnant Ki in the Lower Heater

Symptoms	*Explanation*
Tightness and tension in the arms, shoulders and neck	Obstruction of the Triple Heater Channel
Socially tense/over-cautious	Triple Heater influences wider social relationships and when in harmony reflects extroverted aspects of Fire Element

Stomach Kyo

Symptoms	*Explanation*
Stomach discomfort/lack of appetite and taste/tired in the morning	Stomach-Ki deficiency
Vomiting of clear fluid/cold limbs/loose stools	Stomach-Ki deficiency with Cold
Lack of appetite/dull epigastric pain/fullness after eating/Heat signs	Stomach-Yin deficiency
Overthinking/worry/poor concentration	Pensiveness is the 'emotion' of the Earth Element
Despondent/apathetic	No 'appetite' for life

Stomach Jitsu

Symptoms	*Explanation*
Fullness and swelling in the Stomach/bad breath/lack of appetite	Retention of Food in the Stomach due to stagnant Ki
Belching/'heartburn'/hiccups/vomiting	Stomach Ki rebelling upwards due to stagnant Ki
Burning pain in the Stomach/thirst for cold drinks/hunger/bleeding gums	Fire and Phlegm in the Stomach
Stiffness on the anterior surfaces of the leg	Obstruction of Stomach Channel
Over-thinking/obsessiveness	Pensiveness is the 'emotion' of the Earth Element
Mania/manic depression	Excessive Stomach Heat and Phlegm agitates and clouds the Mind

Large Intestines Kyo

Symptoms	*Explanation*
Loose stools/borborygmi/dull pain in the abdomen/cold limbs	Cold in the Large Intestines, associated with Spleen-Yang deficiency
Haemorrhoids	Spleen-Yang deficiency leads to collapse of Large Intestines
Dry stools/constipation	Lack of fluids in Large Intestines due to general Yin/Blood deficiency
Lack of strength in the thumb	Obstruction of Large Intestines Channel
Disappointment/melancholy	Grief is the emotion of the Metal Element
Unenthusiastic/pessimistic/no 'spirit'	Large Intestines related, through the Lungs, to the Corporeal Soul, source of vitality

Large Intestines Jitsu

Symptoms	*Explanation*
Diarrhoea/mucus in stools/burning anus/abdominal pain	Damp-Heat in the Large Intestines
Constipation with dry stools/burning anus/dry, burning mouth	Heat in the Large Intestines
Swelling in the lower Hara	Dampness in the Large Intestines
Remorse/depression	Grief is the emotion of the Metal Element
Worry which cannot be released	Inability to 'let go'

PART 3

SHIATSU DIAGNOSIS

This section deals with systematic methods for assessing levels of health and disharmony. This enables us to build up a picture of the recipient's constitution and condition, so that we can deduce the underlying cause of their disharmony and decide upon the optimum mode of treatment.

The *Nan Ching* (Chapter 61, p.43) suggests a general approach including some or all of the following procedures:

1. Look at and watch the patient.
2. Listen to and smell the patient.
3. Ask the patient questions.
4. Touch the patient.

Chapter 17

Looking Diagnosis

Immediately the client comes into sight we can get an overall impression of them. We can discern their constitutional body type; see whether or not there is a general Fullness or Emptiness in the upper or lower half of their body; make deductions from colour hues on the face, facial markings, blemishes and other visible features. With experience, these can be discerned at a glance.

CONSTITUTIONAL BODY TYPES

Generally an 'excess' body will tend to have tight musculature, compared to a 'deficient' type body which will have soft flesh and poor circulation.

The following presents archetypes within the Five Elements, although we must realize that pure archetypes are rare, and most people are made up of a combination of several Element types.

Water – Soft features. Often dark or bluish complexion. Tends to be lazy, slow and adaptable.

Wood – Hard, tight and strong musculature. Greenish or purplish complexion. Organized, possibly tense. Sudden rigid movement.

Fire – Fine pointed features. Wide forehead and high cheekbones. Red complexion. Sometimes nervous. Adventurous.

Earth – Heavy set, often flaccid. Tendency to be overweight. Sallow, yellow complexion. Slow moving, calm and practical.

Metal – Broad shouldered, but often hollow-chested and lean. White, pale complexion. Careful in movement, enjoying stillness. Rational and slightly melancholic.

POLARITY OF FULL OR EMPTY

A person may present an overall picture of Fullness manifesting as predominant *Jitsu* in the body, or they may present a sense of Emptiness by appearing predominantly *Kyo*. With a predominantly Jitsu or Kyo person it is sometimes possible to see a discrepancy between the upper and lower half of the body. This requires a trained eye, but is something which comes very quickly with practice. Obviously it is clearer if the discrepancy is extreme. Below are some exaggerated possibilities plus broad principles for re-establishing harmony (based on author's clinical observations).

A. Predominantly *Jitsu* with upper body more Jitsu than lower body

General approach: dispersal techniques over entire body, concentrating more on upper half. Find most Kyo area/Channel in lower body and tonify (reaction is often rapid).

B. Predominantly *Jitsu* with lower body more Jitsu than upper body

General approach: dispersal techniques over entire body, concentrating more on lower half. Find most Kyo area/Channel in upper body and tonify (reaction is often rapid, though slower than A).

Fig. 17.1: Right Predominantly Jitsu, upper body more Jitsu than lower

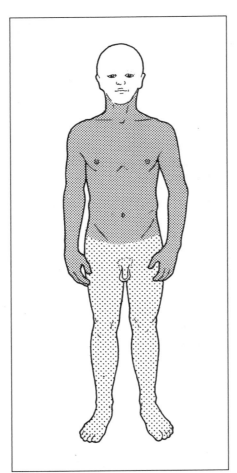

Fig. 17.2: Far right Predominantly Jitsu, lower body more Jitsu than upper

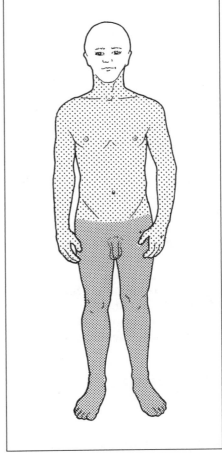

General approach: find most Kyo area/Channel in upper body and tonify (reaction is often considerably slower than Jitsu condition).

C. Predominantly *Kyo* with upper body more Kyo than lower body

General approach: find most Kyo area/Channel in lower body and tonify. This condition generally indicates the weakest condition of the Hara. Therefore holding and tonifying the Hara is effective (reaction usually slow).

D. Predominantly *Kyo* with lower body more Kyo than upper body

Remember that generally, Kyo should be tonified before Jitsu is dispersed. However, sometimes it is necessary to first disperse some Jitsu to reveal the underlying Kyo. This often applies in examples A and B above.

Occasionally you see a major discrepancy between front and back, so that the anterior of the trunk is very Kyo, while the back is Jitsu, or vice versa. Front Jitsu/back Kyo relates to a person who desperately wants to appear strong and able to cope, but whose actual energy reserves are

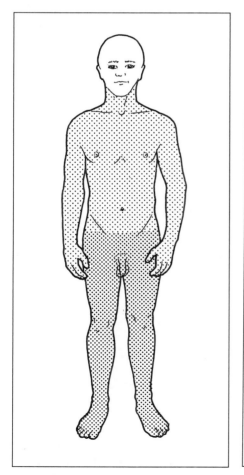
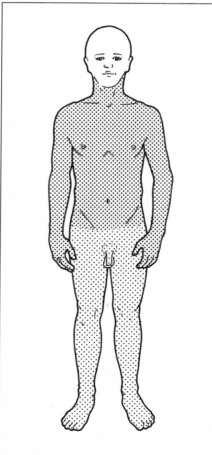

Fig. 17.3: Far left Predominantly Kyo, upper body more Kyo than lower

Fig. 17.4: Left Predominantly Kyo, lower body more Kyo than upper

very limited. These people need tonification on their back and extensive work on their hara. Back Jitsu/front Kyo can indicate a timid, nervous person. Tonification of the Kidney Channel in the chest, plus general tonification of the Hara is very beneficial. Bear in mind that it may require patience to have the receiver feel secure enough to open their Hara to you.

Left/right discrepancies are much more likely when structural imbalances, previous injury or dis-eased organ pathology are present. First check whether the structural imbalance is a skeletal discrepancy, such as a shorter bone on one side of the body, or energetic. If it is not a fixed skeletal problem then tonification of the Kyo channels on the Kyo side is required. The Gall Bladder Channel is often involved.

THE FACE

Complexion Because the Stomach is the source of body fluids, a complexion which is dull or dry looking indicates depleted Stomach Ki, whereas strong Ki is reflected in a clear and moist complexion.

Colour
White – General deficiency and Cold
Red – Heat
Yellow – Spleen deficiency and/or Dampness
Green – Liver disharmony, internal cold or pain
Black Blue – Cold, pain or Kidney disease

Face Areas There are numerous sources of literature exhibiting considerable differences in the correspondences associated with areas on the face. Fig. 17.5 illustrates those areas of facial correspondences born out by our clinical experience.

FACIAL DIAGNOSTIC AREAS

Kidneys Located in the area directly beneath the eyes. Dark rings under the eyes generally indicate weakness of Kidney function. Puffiness indicates Kidney-Yang deficiency. Sunken red hollows may indicate Kidney-Yin deficiency. The condition of the Kidneys may also be revealed through their close link with the ears; redness of the ears often indicates the presence of Heat in the Kidneys.

Liver Located between the eyebrows. Furrows between the eyebrows indicate long-term Liver Ki stagnation. A red patch here indicates Liver-Heat or

Liver-Fire.

Corresponds to the eyelids. Redness of the eyelids may indicate Heat in **Gall Bladder**
the Gall Bladder.

Located on the tip of the nose. A swollen tip indicates a weak Heart **Heart**
function. A red swollen tip may indicate Heat in the Heart.

Located on the inside corner of the eye socket, on the temples and on the **Spleen**
upper bridge of the nose. Darkness and discoloration on the inside
corner of the eye socket indicates Spleen weakness. Yellow discoloration
on the upper bridge of the nose and temples indicates weakness in the
Spleen's transformative function. A vertical line crossing the upper
bridge of the nose between the eyes also indicates long-standing Spleen
disharmony.

Located midway along the bridge of the nose and on the upper lip. A **Stomach**
yellow discoloration indicates weakness in the Stomach's digestive
function. A slight swelling of the upper lip may also indicate a Stomach
disharmony. Dryness and cracking of the upper lip may indicate
Stomach-Yin deficiency.

Located on the cheeks. A white discoloration indicates Lung-Ki and or **Lungs**
-Yang deficiency; a red discoloration may indicate Lung-Yin deficiency
or -Heat.

Corresponds to the nostrils. Redness of the nostrils indicates Heat in the **Bronchi**
bronchii.

Corresponds to the lower lip and the area around the base of the jaw. **Large Intestines**
Red skin eruptions in this area may indicate Damp-Heat in the Large
Intestines. Swelling of the lower lip may indicate weakness in the Large
Intestines' eliminative function, and therefore constipation. Dryness
may indicate a lack of body fluids in the intestines.

Located in the area around the mouth, between the nose and the chin. In **Reproductive Organs**
women, a purple discoloration in this area may indicate stagnation of Ki
in the Lower Heater, causing pre-menstrual tension and menstrual pain.
Red skin eruption in this area indicates Damp-Heat in the reproductive
organs.

Nervous System   Located on the forehead. Bearing in mind the person's age, a large number of vertical lines may indicate weakness in the function of the nervous system.

Please note that these associations are very generalized and should be considered only in the light of a more general diagnosis, taking into account information provided by the patient's symptoms and tongue. For example, while red cheeks may indicate Heat in the Lungs, it may equally indicate overall Yin deficiency. Although we have linked the lips to the Stomach and Large Intestines, they may also reflect the condition of the Spleen as the 'Spleen opens onto the lips'. Despite the fact that the 'Kidneys open into the ears', the ears can also show the condition of the entire body.

Eyes   The eyes reflect the state of the mind (Shen) and Essence (Jing). If the state of Mind and Essence is strong, the eyes will be clear and bright. If the Mind is disturbed and the Essence is weak, the eyes will be lustreless and cloudy.

Fig. 17.5: The face

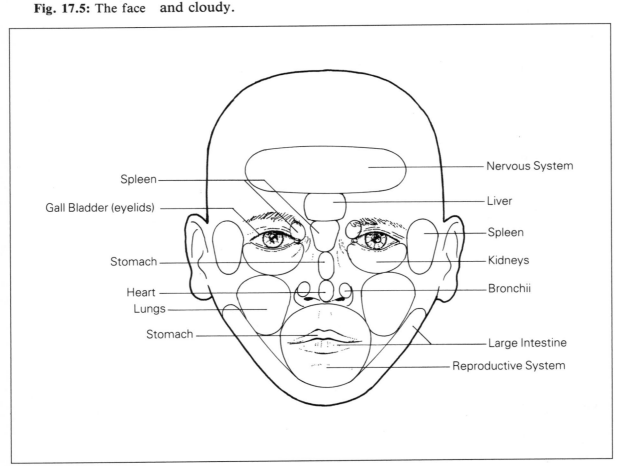

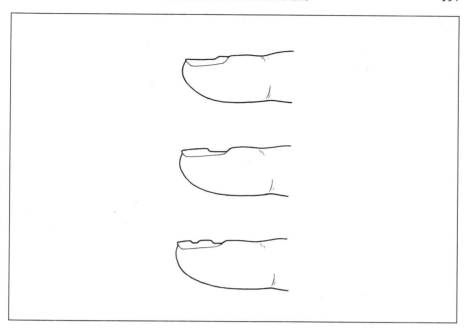

Fig. 17.6: The nails

(a) Vitality better recently

(b) Vitality worse recently

(c) Fluctuating vitality

NAILS

Moist and healthy nails reflect the vitality of the Liver. If there is deficient Liver-Blood to nourish the nails, they will become dry, dark, indented and possibly cracked. Concave nails reflect a chronic Lung Kyo condition.

A sudden decrease in Liver-Blood will result in a sudden decrease in nail thickness, allowing us to establish when the deficiency occurred, provided it was within the previous twelve months (fingernails take six months to grow; toenails take approximately twelve months). Conversely, restoration of nail thickness will tell us that Liver-Blood has been restored.

TOES AND FINGERS

Longstanding Kyo or Jitsu distortion in the Channels can often be seen to produce lateral or medial deviation of the toe into which the Channel flows. The fingers tend not to have these deviations because they are not confined and restricted like the toes.

A lateral deviation indicates Jitsu whereas medial deviation indicates Kyo. Jitsu can also cause a toe to cross over another toe, whereas Kyo can result in a toe dropping and crossing *under* another toe.

Spleen Kyo and Liver Jitsu could cause lateral deviation of the big toe, especially if there is chronic Spleen Kyo *and* Liver Jitsu. Medial deviation of the big toe and lateral deviation of the fifth toe is unlikely, due to the pressure of shoes against them.

A weak looking toe or finger with a narrow 'waist' indicates constitutional weakness in the Channels flowing into it.

Very chronic constipation commonly results in stiffness of the index fingers.

Fig. 17.7: Toes and fingers

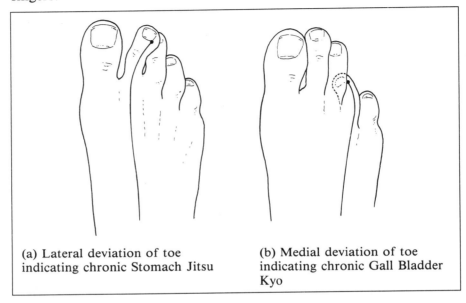

(a) Lateral deviation of toe indicating chronic Stomach Jitsu

(b) Medial deviation of toe indicating chronic Gall Bladder Kyo

Fig. 17.8: Finger with narrow 'waist'

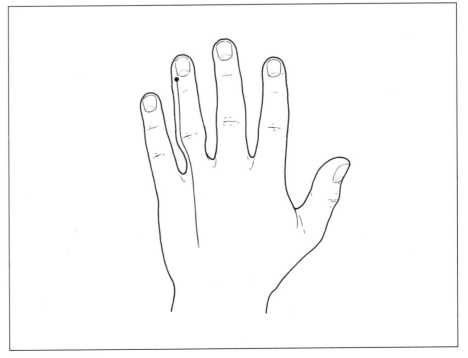

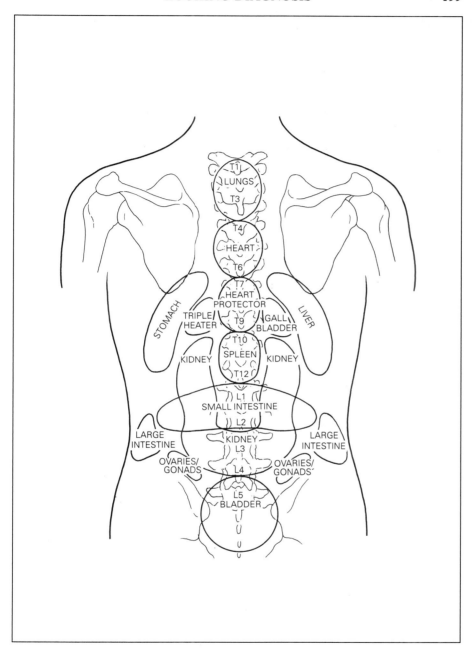

Fig. 17.9: Back Organ Correspondences by area

BACK DIAGNOSIS

With the recipient lying prone, relative Jitsu and Kyo areas can be seen. Do not adjust the receiver's clothing because folds and creases often highlight areas of imbalance. Jitsu will be seen to stand out whereas Kyo will seem flatter or more depressed than normal. With practice, marked skeletal imbalances such as excessive thoracic roundness (or kyphosis) cease to be a distraction. You might for example mistake thoracic kyphosis as Heart Protector Jitsu. As with touch, try to discern Kyo/Jitsu by the absence or presence of vitality.

Figure 17.9 shows the back area correspondences.

Kyo/Jitsu can also be seen along the Channels. For example, Bladder Jitsu is really noticeable where it runs either side of the spinal column, in the buttock and along the back of the legs.

It is easier if the receiver wears plain-coloured clothing to avoid distractions. If you cannot see any obvious Kyo/Jitsu, covering the receiver with a white sheet will often highlight it. (Do explain to them first, or they may think the procedure rather strange.)

Chapter 18

Touch Diagnosis

Touch Diagnosis is the most important ingredient in the Shiatsu health assessment because the entire technique and purpose of Shiatsu is to touch. Therefore it is only natural that touch should be the primary diagnostic tool.

CHANNEL DIAGNOSIS

Excess or deficient Ki within the Channels can be felt as a Jitsu or Kyo quality as we apply Shiatsu technique to the Channels. The qualities of both Jitsu and Kyo have been discussed already on pp.17–19. In short, if the receiver feels your touch as dull sensation, dull soreness or ache, this indicates a Kyo condition. Sharp sensation such as sharp pain indicates a Jitsu condition. Each Channel will exhibit some areas of Jitsu and some of Kyo, although one will predominate. A total rebalance of Ki within the Channels could be achieved by working each Channel along its entire surface pathway, tonifying or dispersing Kyo and Jitsu wherever it is located. However, this would be a long, laborious process. Alternatively, each Channel could be stretched in the arms and legs using the techniques detailed in Chapter 6.

A Jitsu condition will feel hard, but with an elastic feel of resistance, whereas a Kyo condition will feel flabby, weak and often stiff if deeply penetrated. For maximum effectiveness, treatment can be administered to the most Kyo and the most Jitsu Channels.

HARA DIAGNOSIS

There are several facets to Hara diagnosis useful to Shiatsu practitioners.

Zen Shiatsu Hara Diagnosis

This method enables us to find the most Kyo and most Jitsu Channels more quickly than direct palpation or stretching of the Channels. Figure

Fig. 18.1: Zen Shiatsu
Hara diagnosis areas

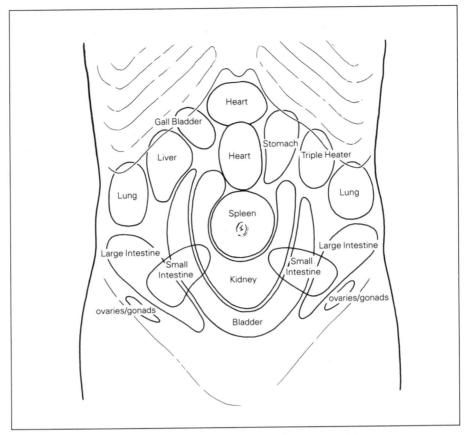

18.1 gives a map of the twelve abdominal areas which relate to the twelve major Channels. Kyo or Jitsu found in these areas will reflect the energetic state of the corresponding Channels.

There are three methods of applying this system, namely:

● Deep Touch Method
● Light Touch Method
● No Touch Method

The *deep touch method* requires moderately deep pressure for the purpose of locating pain, discomfort, tension, strength or weakness of the abdominal muscles, pulsing of blood vessels or lumps. Any of these observations can indicate by inference the interplay of Kyo/Jitsu. A sense of *reaction* indicates Jitsu, whereas *lack of reaction* signifies Kyo. Be careful to discount matter or gas in the intestines. If you feel any other lumps, especially if they feel like 'cauliflower', gently suggest that the client has it medically examined, if they have not already done so.

The *light touch method* is quicker and free from distractions by the abdominal contents. The diagnostic areas are scanned with the lightest

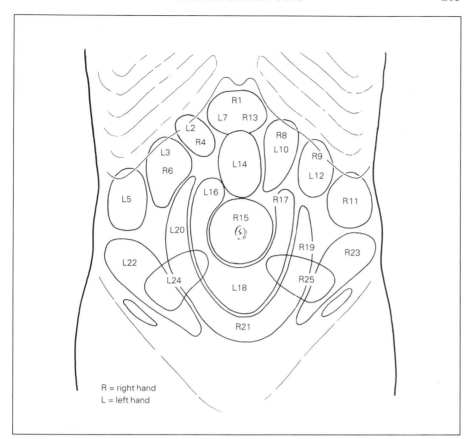

Fig. 18.2: Sequence for two hand scanning of the Hara; this sequence is used for both the deep touch and light touch methods

touch using the fingertips of both hands, in the sequence illustrated in Figure 18.2. This sequence enables each area to be contacted twice, thus allowing a constant comparison with an adjacent area or with the Heart area.

Once the most Kyo and most Jitsu areas have been discovered they can be checked by first holding the *Jitsu* area, then holding the *Kyo* area with the other hand. If the assessment is correct, there will be a definite feeling of connection and reaction between the two areas. In particular, the Jitsu area will feel like it is 'opening' or 'sinking'. If you get no reaction, try holding another Kyo area. Because the Jitsu area is easier to find, it is less likely to have been incorrectly diagnosed. Continue in this manner until you get a definite reaction.

This is a very subtle and consequently a very subjective approach, which works better if you trust your first impression. The longer you think about it and the more you try to cross check it, the more your analytical faculties will interfere with your sensitivity. This method is very 'Zen', in that the less you struggle for an answer, the more likely the answer will come.

Making a quick decision is also necessary in this instance, because the more you pad around on the Hara, the more likely you are to initiate an energetic change, and therefore arrive at a reading which is modified by your touch.

The *no touch method* involves passing your palms over each area at a distance of 2–4 inches. For this method, you need to be sensitive to the etheric field of Ki around the body, which although sounding esoteric, is in fact easier and more tangible for many people than discerning Kyo/Jitsu through touch. As you move your hand slowly you can feel sensations of heat, cold, or what feels like an updraught of wind. Heat and/or an updraught of wind indicate Jitsu. Cold often indicates Kyo. A feeling of uniformity, like riding on a carpet of air, is a sign of natural health. Feelings of an empty hole in this 'carpet' indicate Kyo. This method, when mastered, enables you quickly to narrow down the entire energetic distortions to the deepest underlying Kyo deficiency.

It is common for the Kyo/Jitsu reading to be different on the Hara compared to the reading on the Back. This does not mean that each method is in contradiction to the other, but that they each illustrate different depths of the receiver's energetic imbalances. The Back is usually considered to display more chronic imbalances whereas the Hara indicates more acute imbalances. With experience, however, the Hara reading can indicate the deepest underlying imbalance. Whether you treat according to the Hara or the Back will depend on which level of the recipient's problem you wish to tackle on that particular occasion, and to some extent on which of your senses you believe to be the most reliable and clear; the visual or the tactile.

Five Reflex Hara Diagnosis

This system is less precise, but can be used to indicate broadly marked imbalances in any of the Five Elements. Indications in this system tend to manifest on a much more physical level in the form of 'abdominal masses'. Abdominal masses that move under fingertip pressure indicate stagnation of Ki. Hard masses that do not move indicate stasis of Blood.

Note that all the correspondences along the vertical midline are similar to the Zen Shiatsu system (see Fig. 18.3).

Other Indications from the Hara

● The upper Hara just below the xiphoid process and Directing Vessel-15 should be looser than the rest. If if feels hard and knotted it indicates a constraint of Heart and Lung Ki. The lower Hara below the umbilicus and around Directing Vessel-6 should feel elastic but firmer and tighter than the rest. If it feels soft and flabby it indicates a weakness of the Original Ki which resides between the Kidneys to activate all physiological functions and to provide heat for digestion. To strengthen the lower Hara and Original Ki, tonification should be applied to the Kidney and Triple Heater channels. (The Triple Heater is the 'avenue' for the Original Ki, distributing it to all the organs and ultimately to all the channels.)

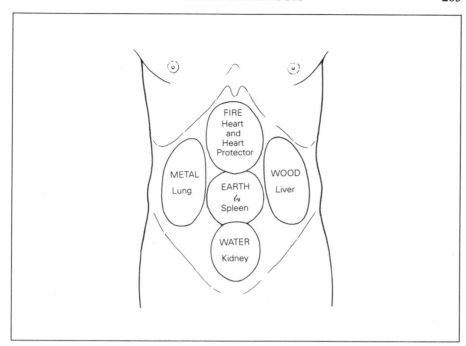

Fig. 18.3: The 'Five Reflex' abdominal areas

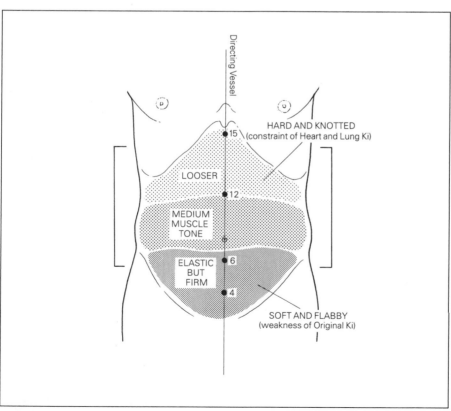

Fig. 18.4: Directing Vessel-6, -12, -15

The mid Hara above the umbilicus, around Directing Vessel-12, should have less tightness than Directing Vessel-6, but be firmer than Directing Vessel-15 (see Fig. 18.4).

- A painful Hara is a sign of deficient Spleen and Kidneys.
- The Directing Vessel line should be slightly depressed and lower than the Kidney and Stomach Channel lines (like a shallow valley). If it is raised above the Kidney and Stomach line, and especially distended around Directing Vessel-12, a weak Hara is indicated.
- Tension or spasm in the abdominal muscles when the Hara is in a relaxed position signifies deficient Kidney (and sometimes Spleen) Ki.
- An umbilicus which is close to the surface indicates a weaker Hara than if the umbilicus is deeply set. Strong pulsing around the umbilicus indicates deficient Spleen Ki. If the pulse is not central within the umbilicus, postural irregularities may be present. For example, if the pulse is to the left of the umbilicus, check for tightness and constriction on the left side of the torso.
- If there is pulsing below the sternum, which reaches down to the umbilicus, Heart and Kidney deficiency is indicated.

THE BACK TRANSPORTING POINTS

The Back Transporting Points are also known as Yu Points (Japanese) or Shu Points (Chinese). They are useful in diagnosis because they become tender on pressure when their associated Organ is ailing.

They are also very useful in the treatment of chronic disease. In addition they can be used to treat the sense organs of the corresponding visceral organs. The specific action of each Back Transporting Point is given under the discussion of Tsubos on p.229. Fig. 18.5 gives the location and associated Organ of these points.

THE FRONT COLLECTING POINTS

The Front Collecting Points are also known as Bo Points (Japanese) or Mu Points (Chinese). Like the Back Transporting Points, these points become tender when their associated Organ is ailing.

In treatment they have a regulating effect upon the internal Organs. They are useful in both acute and chronic dysfunction although they are more often used in acute cases.

Figure 18.6 gives the location and associated organ of these Points.

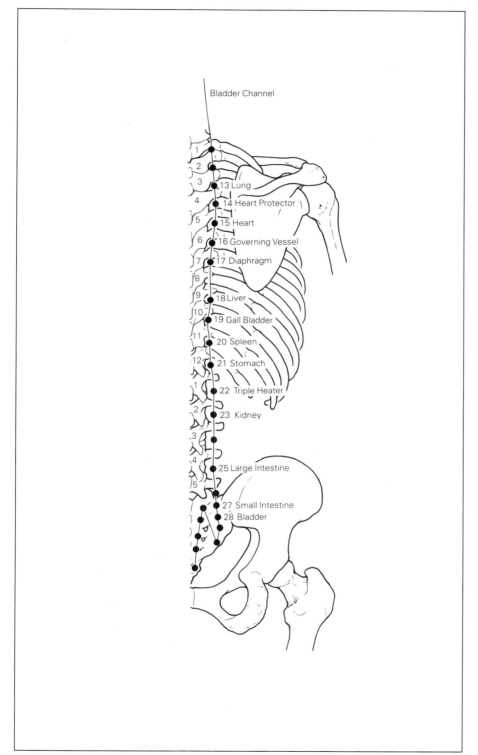

Fig. 18.5: The Back Transporting Points

Fig. 18.6: The Front
Collecting Points

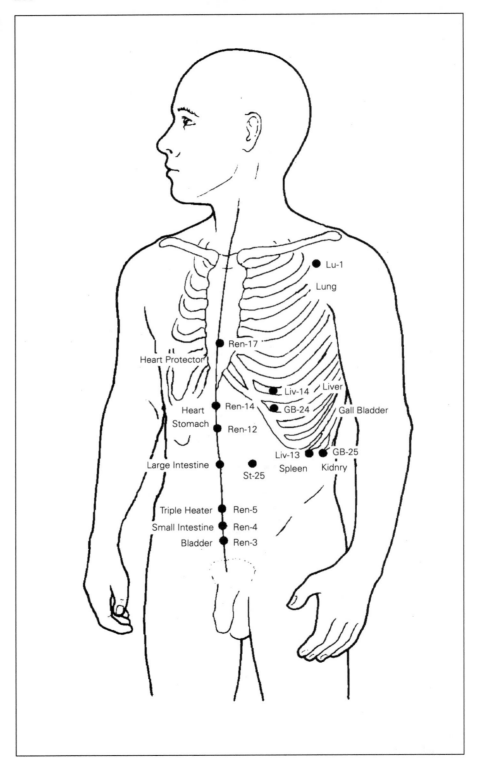

Chapter 19

Diagnosis Through Listening and Smelling

The relatively subtle diagnostic techniques of listening and smelling provide us with information gleaned from the sound of a client's voice and breathing, and the natural odour of their body.

The voice can be a fascinating source of insight into the emotional disposition of an individual. Like the emotions, the different sounds of the voice are categorized according to the Five Elements, and therefore offer information about the client's constitutional make-up. This means that the condition of Elements and Organs to which they point reveals potential, not necessarily actual, energetic problems. The sound of the voice should not generally be relied upon to provide us with information regarding the client's current physical condition.

The Sound of the Voice

When attempting to discern the underlying sound of the voice, one must focus one's attention away from both the subject matter being spoken of as well as the style or accent of the voice. This may take practice: one can first listen to the voices of fellow students and friends with the eyes closed, as they read aloud subject matter which will not distract.

The Kidneys give depth to the voice. However, the Water Element in disharmony will produce a groaning sound, especially discernible at the end of words and phrases. It may reveal a tendency towards feeling threatened or insecure.

The Liver gives the voice a sense of authority. When the Wood Element is affected there will be the presence of a shout in the voice. Alternatively, the person's voice may possess a clipped quality. A propensity towards feeling frustrated and angry is naturally indicated.

Ruling the tongue, the Heart ensures that words are well articulated. Speech impediments such as stuttering often reflect an energetic imbalance of the Heart. The Heart also gives a sense of buoyancy to the voice. When there is a tremulous quality to the voice, traditionally described as a Laugh, a problem with the Fire Element may be indicated. The person is likely to be prone to over-excitement or anxiety.

The Spleen gives a singing quality to the voice. A voice that has a singing sound which overrides all other qualities means that a disharmony of the Earth Element is probable. The person may tend to worry a lot.

Finally, the Lungs give strength to the voice. A voice which is weak may indicate Lung deficiency. Moreover, an underlying weeping sound in the voice may point to a problem with the Metal Element, and reveal a corresponding presence of sadness or Grief.

Finally, it must be stressed that, just as an individual possesses a number of predominating emotions, a voice may contain more than one predominating sound. Thus, it is by no means uncommon to be able to discern two, or even three, main sounds in the voice.

In general, a loud voice indicates the presence of a Full condition, whereas a quiet one reflects an Empty condition. In the same way, breathing which sounds feeble and faint points to an Empty condition. A wheezing sound reflects the presence of Dampness or Phlegm in the Lungs.

The Odour The odour is more difficult than the voice to diagnose in the context of Shiatsu Therapy, simply because the receiver remains clothed. However, practitioners who train their nose will still be able to smell the natural odour of a clothed person. This odour should not be confused with the body odour produced by perspiration. It is more subtle and is most present around the chest and upper back.

A putrid, stagnant odour indicates a Kidney disharmony. A rancid, sour odour indicates a Liver imbalance (or Retention of Food). A faint scorched smell, like freshly ironed linen, points to either a Heart disharmony or the presence of Heat. A sickly sweet or 'Fragrant' odour reflects a problem with the Spleen. A rotten, musty odour indicates either a Lung disharmony or the presence of Phlegm in the body.

SOUND AND ODOUR: FIVE ELEMENT RELATIONSHIPS

	Water/ Kidney	Wood/ Liver	Fire/ Heart	Earth/ Spleen	Metal/ Lung
Sound	Groan	Shout/ clipped	Laugh/ tremulous	Sing	Weep
Odour	Putrid	Rancid	Scorched	Sweet/ Fragrant	Rotten/ musty

Chapter 20

Pulse Diagnosis

Reading the pulse according to Oriental Medicine provides information about the patient's entire constitution and condition. It accurately reflects the state of the Ki, the Blood, of Yin and Yang in the body, and of the internal Organs. Along with tongue diagnosis, it has traditionally been the most important tool of health assessment.

Pulse diagnosis in its complete form is very complex, some of which is not applicable in Shiatsu practice. What we will present here is a simplified approach.

Like Hara diagnosis, pulse diagnosis is relatively more subjective than other forms of diagnosis. It requires considerable skill in discerning the subtle distinctions between different types of pulse. Even the simple form outlined below will require additional supervised instruction and a great deal of practice to master. It should also be remembered that pulse diagnosis is often subject to short-term influences which may obscure an accurate reading of the patient's true underlying condition. Temporary states of depletion and emotional upset will be reflected in the pulse.

METHOD OF PULSE-TAKING

Ensure that the patient's arm is horizontal. It should not be held at a level higher than that of the heart. The practitioner should use their first three fingers to feel the patient's pulse, which is located along the radial artery just below the wrist.

The left-hand pulse is generally more indicative of the state of the patient's Blood. It is usually slightly stronger in men. The right-hand pulse is generally more indicative of the patient's Ki, and is usually slightly stronger in women.

A pulse which is 'gentle' and resilient and lacks any feeling of roughness indicates strong Stomach Ki. As the first Organ of digestion, the Stomach is the origin of Ki, Blood and Body Fluids, and therefore representative of the Ki as a whole. A pulse which is regular, neither strong nor weak, and maintains a consistent quality is said to have

Fig. 20.1: Pulse-taking

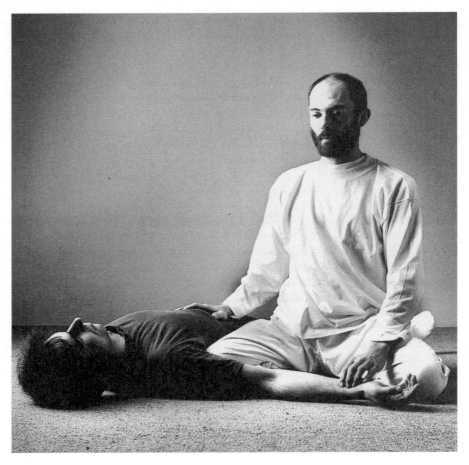

'spirit', and reflects a healthy condition of the Heart, Blood and Mind.
   A pulse which can be clearly felt at a deep level is considered to have 'root', and reflects the condition of the Kidneys and Essence.

12 MAIN PULSE QUALITIES

1. Superficial/Float-
ing Pulse

To feel this pulse the practitioner need only place their fingers lightly on the patient's artery.

- Indicates an External condition, as Ki rises to the surface to defend the Interior;
  Superficial and Tight: External Wind-Cold;
  Superficial and Wiry: External Wind-Heat.
- A pulse which is both Superficial and Empty at a deep level indicates Yin deficiency.

This pulse is opposite to a Superficial pulse and requires a deep pressure to reach it.
2. Deep Pulse

- Indicates an Internal condition, one that mainly involves the Yin Organs.

The normal rate of the pulse varies according to age and constitutional type. The following table gives rough approximations of a norm:
3. Slow Pulse

Age (in years)	Rate (beats per min)
1–4	90 plus
4–10	84
10–16	78
16–35	74
35–50	70
50 and over	68

A rate which is 10–20 beats slower than those indicated in the table may be considered a Slow pulse.

- A Slow pulse indicates the presence of Cold;
  Slow and Empty: indicates Cold generated from Yang deficiency;
  Slow and Full: indicates Cold of an Excess nature, usually the result of external invasion.

A pulse which is 10–20 beats faster than the normal rates indicated in the table may be considered a Rapid pulse.
4. Rapid Pulse

- A Rapid pulse indicates the presence of Heat;
  Rapid and Empty: indicates Heat generated from Yin deficiency;
  Rapid and Full: indicates Heat of an Excess nature.

This pulse may feel big but has no strength to it; it is soft to the touch.
5. Empty Pulse

- Indicates Ki-deficiency.

This pulse feels big, full and relatively hard.
6. Full Pulse

- Indicates a Full condition;
  Full and Rapid: indicates Excess Heat;
  Full and Slow: indicates Excess Cold.

This pulse feels very smooth and slippery, and feels like something sliding through oil.
7. Slippery Pulse

- Usually indicates Dampness, Phlegm or Retention of Food; can also reflect pregnancy.

8. Choppy Pulse   This pulse feels slightly rough to the touch, like a toothbrush. It can also mean a pulse which changes frequently in rate and quality.

- Indicates Blood deficiency and occasionally depletion of Body Fluids.

9. Thready/Fine/ Thin Pulse   This pulse is very fine, like a piece of thread.

- Indicates Blood deficiency and occasionally Dampness with Ki-deficiency.

10. Tight Pulse   This pulse feels hard and taut, like a twisted rope.

- Indicates a Cold condition;
  Tight and Superficial: indicates External Cold;
  Tight and Deep: indicates Internal Cold.
- A Tight pulse may also reflect pain.

11. Wiry Pulse   This pulse is thinner, harder and more taut than the Tight pulse. It is often likened to a guitar string.

- Usually indicates Liver-Ki stagnation; can also reflect pain or the presence of Phlegm.

12. Weak Pulse   This pulse is both deep and soft.

- Indicates Yang deficiency.

Chapter 21

Tongue Diagnosis

Tongue diagnosis is a very accurate and reliable way of assessing the patient's condition. It is less subjective than pulse diagnosis, may be mastered more quickly, and is generally not subject to temporary changes in the patient's condition.

It is important to have an adequate amount of natural light to see the tongue properly for detailed diagnosis. When this is not available, a small torch should be used. The patient should not have taken food or drink in the half-hour prior to observation of the tongue.

THE SHAPE OF THE TONGUE BODY

- Thin and pale: Blood deficiency
- Thin and red: Yin deficiency

Thin

- Swollen and pale: Spleen and/or Kidney Yang deficiency causing Dampness
- Swollen and red: Damp Heat

Swollen

- Spleen Ki deficiency

Teeth marks around edge

- Heat in the Heart

Long

- Short and pale: Spleen Yang deficiency causing Internal Cold
- Short and red: Yin deficiency or Excess Heat

Short

- Cracks generally indicate Yin deficiency or Excess Heat
- Short horizontal cracks: Yin deficiency

Cracked

Fig. 21.1: Tongue areas

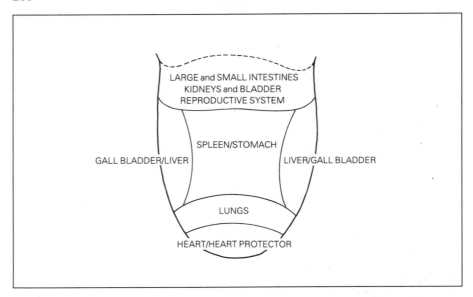

- Short horizontal cracks on the sides of the tongue: Spleen-Ki deficiency
- A long, deep crack along the mid-line extending to the tip: constitutional Heart weakness
- A crack along the mid-line which does not extend to the tip: Stomach and/or Kidney Yin deficiency

Peeled
- Yin deficiency

Quivering
- Quivering and pale: Spleen Ki deficiency
- Quivering and red: Heat generating Internal Wind

Rolled
- Tip rolled under: Excess Heat
- Tip rolled over: Heat from Yin deficiency

Ulcerated
- Heart Fire

THE COLOUR OF THE TONGUE BODY

The colour of the tongue body indicates the condition of the Blood.

Pale
- Pale, swollen and wet: Yang deficiency
- Pale and dry: Blood deficiency

- Red: Heat   **Red**
- Red, dry and without coating: Heat from Yin deficiency
- Red and wet: Heat and Dampness
- Red and shiny: Stomach and/or Kidney Yin deficiency
- Scarlet red: Lung and/or Heart Yin deficiency
- Red spots: localized Heat
- Red with large red spots: Heat with stagnant Blood

- Purple: stagnation of Ki or Blood   **Purple**
- Reddish purple: Ki/Blood stagnation with Heat
- Bluish-purple: Ki/Blood stagnation with Cold

- Internal Cold   **Blue**

TONGUE COATING

Whereas the shape and colour of the tongue body more commonly reflect the condition of the Blood and Yin Organs, the tongue coating is particularly indicative of the state of the Yang organs, especially the Stomach.

It is in fact the Stomach which produces the tongue coating. A certain amount of Dampness is left over from the digestion of food, and travels upwards to the tongue. It is therefore normal to have a thin, white coating.

A tongue coating which is thicker than normal indicates the presence of an Internal or External pathogenic factor. An absence of tongue coating indicates Yin deficiency.

- Cold and Dampness in the Middle Heater   **White and Thick**

- Normal body colour: External Wind-Cold   **White, Thick and**
- Pale body colour: Internal Cold and Dampness   **Wet**

- Retention of Food from Yang deficiency   **White, Thick and Greasy**

- External Wind-Heat   **Thin Yellow**

- Internal Damp-Heat   **Thick Yellow**

Dirty Yellow   ● Damp-Heat in the Stomach and Intestines

Yellow, Sticky or   ● Phlegm-Heat
Greasy

Grey and Wet   ● Cold-Damp in the Spleen

Grey and Dry   ● Excess Heat

Chapter 22

Questioning and Case-Taking

Asking relevant questions gives a general impression of the history and lifestyle of the recipient, as well as information about the level of health or disease amongst blood relations. This information will help us to determine the underlying cause of their disharmony and will often indicate their prognosis.

For example, if a 40-year-old man presents with symptoms which suggest heart problems, and questions reveal that his father, grandfather and brother all died from heart failure before they reached the age of 45, then a major hereditary or familial problem is indicated. A poor prognosis suggests itself unless a common factor which can be treated is identified. It may be that the whole family has always subsisted on fried eggs and sugar, with a total aversion to exercise. The treatment aim is then obvious, but he may not have given this information had you not asked.

The answers to your questions, along with your observations on all levels as described throughout this chapter, will constitute the framework for a case history. Not all questions need to be answered in every case, and others may need to be added. The most important consideration is to 'communicate' with your clients, rather than interrogate them.

Of course, by simply finding and treating the most Kyo and Jitsu Channels, the energetic distortions can be positively affected. However, the case history questionnaire enables us to find out from which level of pathology the distortions arise. This means that we can assess the root cause and prognosis, and offer supplementary advice on such things as exercise, diet and lifestyle where applicable.

A CASE HISTORY FORMAT

Name: D.o.b.   Date:
Address: Male/Female:
Tel: Day: Evening:

Subjective Assessment (verbal information given by the client)

Reasons for seeking treatment
This usually reflects the symptoms most urgently in need of attention from the recipient's perspective.

Medical history
This may provide a clue to current symptoms; operations or accident trauma may have weakened or obstructed certain Channels due to the removal of organs or the build up of scar tissue, therefore causing pain local to the scar tissue, or elsewhere along the affected Channel.

The medical history may also indicate how chronic a condition is. If the client comes to be treated for eczema and questioning reveals they were born with it, and have been extensively treated using many different approaches from birth onwards, then we can conclude that it is very chronic and deep seated, and requires extensive treatment to alleviate.

Medical history of family
Include parents, grandparents, brothers and sisters. This may highlight a hereditary influence or a familial pattern such as described in the introduction to this chapter.

Medication
Past: Medical drugs may produce side effects which confuse the diagnosis or produce more extreme reactions to treatment.

Fatigue patterns
Feeling drowsy after meals indicates Spleen-Ki deficiency.
Extreme lethargy with a feeling of cold is characteristic of Kidney-Yang deficiency.

Sleep patterns
Any problems relating to sleep can result from excess Yang, Yin deficiency or Blood deficiency. However, difficulty in getting to sleep is usually due to excess Yang.

Light sleep when one wakes at the slightest sound is more often due to Blood deficiency.
Restless, disturbed sleep relates to Yin deficiency.

Hot/cold
Coldness indicates Yang deficiency.
Feeling hot can result from either excess Yang or Yin deficiency.
Heat from Yin Deficiency is more common at night and in the late afternoon.

Perspiration
Excessive perspiration can result from both excess Yang and Yin deficiency.
Yin deficiency more commonly causes sweating at night only.
Lack of perspiration may indicate deficient Yang or Cold.

Thirst
Hot conditions are characterized by the desire to drink cold liquids, usually in large volumes.
Cold conditions are characterized by a lack of thirst or the desire to drink warm liquids; usually the Stomach or Spleen is implicated.

Diet and digestion
Empty conditions are usually relieved by eating.
Full conditions are usually aggravated by eating.
Lack of appetite reflects Spleen Ki deficiency.
Constant hunger reflects Heat in the Stomach.
Distension after eating indicates Retention of Food.
Hot conditions create a craving for Cold food.
Cold conditions create a craving for Hot food.
Food fads and extreme dietary philosophies may encourage an inappropriate diet for the individual, often generating symptoms of deficiency.

Alcohol
Excessive alcohol consumption tends to generate Heat in the body and deplete the Yin. It may also give rise to disharmonies of the Liver.

Smoking
Smoking leads to the creation of Heat and Phlegm in the Lungs and Heart. This can lead to lung cancer and heart disease. In our experience, because smoking produces Heat in the Blood, skin problems cannot be resolved until the client ceases to smoke.

Drugs

The majority of 'recreational' drugs are extremely deleterious to the bodymind and seriously injure the Ki, Blood and Essence.

Prolonged use of drugs such as heroin and cocaine generates Heat, consumes the Yin of the Kidneys, Stomach and Heart, and causes Liver-Ki stagnation.

Hallucinogenic drugs and amphetamines particularly weaken the nervous system.

All such drugs disturb the Mind (Shen) and can lead to depression, anxiety, paranoia and aggressive behaviour.

Pain

The assessment of pain is very useful in Shiatsu because it reflects directly the circulation and quantity of Ki in the channels, which can be directly or indirectly influenced by Shiatsu. If the Channels are free from obstruction there is no pain.

Sharp, localized pain, as in Jitsu conditions, can be caused by:

- invasion by external pathogenic factors
- stagnation of Ki, Blood or Phlegm
- obstruction by Phlegm   } obstructing Ki in
- retention of Food   the Channels
- internal Cold or Heat

Dull, empty, less focused pain reflects deficiency conditions, or Kyo within the Channels. It is caused by deficiency of Ki and Blood.

Headaches

The most common type of headache is caused by stress and feels 'tight', like a band around the head, or from the back of the neck towards the eyes. This results from Liver-Ki stagnation and is also often accompanied by nausea.

Another common type of headache is a pounding or throbbing type, often accompanied by a burning sensation in the eyes. This is caused by Liver-Yang rising or Liver-Fire.

Headaches with a deep, boring pain result from Blood deficiency or Blood stagnation.

Headaches on the front of the head are commonly caused by Stomach problems, e.g. Retention of Food, often accompanied by indigestion.

Headaches on the back of the head often involve the Kidneys.

Menstruation

Pre-menstrual tension and pre-menstrual pain both result from stagnation of Liver Ki or Blood.

Pain during the period is usually caused by Heat in the Blood or stagnation of Cold.

Pain and weakness after the period is caused by Blood deficiency.
Heavy periods when the Blood is dark red or bright are caused by Heat in the Blood.
Heavy bleeding when the Blood is pale is caused by Ki deficiency.
Scanty Blood or absence of menstruation is caused by Blood deficiency or stagnation of Blood.
Clots in the menstrual Blood indicate stagnation of Blood.

Bowels
Constipation may be caused by Liver-Ki stagnation, Blood deficiency, Yin deficiency, or Heat.
Loose stools and diarrhoea generally suggest Spleen-Yang or Kidney-Yang deficiency.
Alternating constipation and diarrhoea are typical of Liver Ki invading the Spleen.

Urine
Scanty urination indicates Kidney-Yin deficiency.
Large amounts of pale urine indicate Kidney-Yang deficiency.
Pale urine indicates Cold conditions whereas dark urine indicates Heat.

Objective Assessment (Information you acquire using your senses: seeing, hearing, smelling, touching)

Skin
Skin conditions often point to a condition of the Lungs. However, the following factors can also affect the skin: Heat in the Blood caused by Liver or Stomach Heat; stagnation or deficiency of Liver Blood. These conditions cause dryness, redness, itching and scaling skin. Pus conditions involve Dampness or Phlegm.

Swellings
All abnormal lumps should be checked by a medical doctor if they have not previously been examined, especially if they look or feel like cauliflower, or are growing or changing in any way.
Pitting oedema, called water oedema in Chinese Medicine, results from Kidney Yang deficiency.

Posture
A general sense of strength or weakness, rigidity or openness, depression or optimism, can be observed in the posture.
Differences in the height of each shoulder, or other anomalies are worth checking as they may indicate some distortions in the Channels or skeletal structure. Such distortions may be the cause or the result of dysfunctions within the internal organs.

Constitutional type
See p.191.

Breathing
Shallow breathing can indicate Lung-Ki deficiency.
Wheezing can mean Phlegm in the Lungs.
Constriction in the chest can arise because of Liver Ki stagnation.

Nails
See p.197.

Face
See p.194.

Tongue
See p.215.

Pulse
See p.211.

Hara
See p.201.

Back
See p.199.

Element Correspondences

- **Colour**   (see page 194)
- **Sound**
- **Odour**   (see page 210)
- **Emotion**

Comments
Any other information considered relevant, such as stiffness in specific joints, general attitude of the client, and so on, should be included.

Conclusion (Diagnosis)

A common thread will emerge from the case history which will substantiate the Hara, Back or Pulse diagnosis. Experience gives the practitioner the ability to extract what is relevant, and to narrow down all the presenting factors to reveal the underlying causes of the recipient's condition.

Chapter 23

Case Study Examples

The following case study examples reflect situations when the pathology of the Internal Organs, as explained according to Traditional Oriental Medicine, are *directly* reflected in the Kyo/Jitsu distortion of the Channels related to those Organs. These examples are archetypes of simple clear cut cases when the Channels and their associated Organs align in their dysfunction. As such, they represent examples of very simple, easy to analyse cases. In the clinic, the Channel/Organ relationship is not always so direct.

In practice, the most Kyo and most Jitsu Channels do not *always* reflect the Internal Organ pathology in such an obvious way. For example, if signs indicating Heart Blood Deficiency are present, that does not mean that the Heart Channel will automatically be Kyo. It might be, but no such assumptions should be made. Conversely, where a specific Channel is found to be the most Kyo or the most Jitsu, it does not *necessarily* follow that clear cut Empty or Full pathologies will be found within the Organ related to that Channel.

With sufficient understanding of theory, one can figure out how and why a Channel distortion may seemingly contradict other signs and symptoms, but such understanding is born of extensive clinical experience rather than discerned through reading books. Therefore, always select the most Kyo and most Jitsu Channels by accurately 'reading'/ sensing the body, primarily through Hara or Back diagnosis. In other words, Channels to treat on the Kyo/Jitsu rebalancing level should be selected through sensitivity to Ki at an experiential level, rather than according to deduction at the intellectual level.

CASE No. 1: KIDNEY KYO/LUNG JITSU

A woman in her early fifties comes for treatment complaining of mild asthma, a 'wheezy' chest and difficulty in catching her breath. Further questioning reveals that she is often tired, feels cold and has copious, clear urination. Her pulse is Empty and her tongue pale and slightly swollen.

In terms of Traditional Oriental Medicine, this is an example of the Kidneys failing to grasp Ki from the Lungs. It is confirmed by a Jitsu condition of the Lung Channel together with a Kyo condition of the Kidney Channel.

The client's asthma, chest congestion and difficulty in catching her breath result from a failure of the Lungs to fulfil their function of descending the Ki. As a result, excess Ki accumulates in the Upper Heater to produce what appears to be a Full condition of the Lungs. It is this apparently Full condition which leads to the Jitsu quality of the Lung Channel.

Part of this condition, however, is a failure of the Kidneys to grasp Ki from the Lungs – a problem which arises from Kidney-Yang deficiency. Deficient Kidney-Yang is evident from her tiredness, feelings of cold and copious, clear urination. The Empty pulse and pale, swollen tongue further confirm a Yang deficient condition.

Treatment   Tonifying the Kidney Channel and Tsubos such as Bladder-23 may in itself be enough to rectify this basically Deficient situation. However, dispersal of the Lung Channel may be necessary if the chest is especially congested with Phlegm.
(For details of treating Kidney-Lung disharmony see p.150.)

CASE No. 2: KIDNEY KYO/LIVER JITSU

A man in his early forties comes for treatment complaining of lower back pain, insomnia, frequent headaches and sore, inflamed eyes. Further questioning reveals that he is frequently thirsty and sweats profusely at night. You notice that he is restless and irritable. His pulse has a Floating quality. His tongue is red, has no coating, is peeled at the rear and swollen at the sides.

In terms of Traditional Oriental Medicine, this is an example of a combination of Kidney-Yin deficiency and Liver-Yang rising. It is confirmed by the fact that the Kidney Channel presents as Kyo in condition and the Liver Channel as Jitsu.

Kidney deficiency is evident from the lower back pain. The patient's thirst, night sweats, insomnia and restlessness are clear indicators of Yin-deficiency. Yin-deficiency is also apparent from a red, peeled tongue without coating. The Kidney-Yin is clearly failing to nourish the Liver-Yin and so 'hold down' the Liver-Yang.

The consequent rising Liver-Yang has resulted in headaches, eye inflammation and irritability. Swelling along the sides of the tongue indicates a Full condition of the Liver. A Floating pulse reveals that the body's Yang has risen to the surface because of a depletion of Yin.

This is an example of how Yin/Yang disharmony in the body can create **Treatment** a basically Kyo condition underlying signs of Jitsu. The Excess Yang/Jitsu condition of the Liver stems directly from the deficient Yin/Kyo condition of the Kidney. The priority in treatment, therefore, is to tonify the Kidney Kyo, and so 'bring down' the Liver Jitsu. It may, however, be necessary to disperse the Liver Channel if the patient is suffering acute symptoms (such as headache) caused by Liver Jitsu.
(For details of treating Kidney-Yin deficiency, see p.149; for Liver-Yang rising, see p.156.)

CASE No. 3: HEART JITSU/LUNG KYO

A woman in her late fifties comes for treatment complaining of occasional palpitations, a feeling of oppression and fullness in the chest, breathlessness and a lack of energy. Upon further questioning you learn that several months ago she visited her doctor after experiencing some pains in the chest. Her face is a bright pale colour, her lips are slightly blue and her hands are cold. She also mentions that she is prone to sweating in the day for no apparent reason. Her pulse is Empty; her tongue pale and slightly purple.

In terms of Oriental Medicine, the patient's condition combines an apparently Full pattern of the Heart (stagnation of Heart-Blood), with an Empty pattern of the Lungs (Lung-Ki deficiency). However, the underlying condition of the Heart is one of deficiency, producing a situation that calls for careful application of tonification and dispersal.

Symptoms of stagnant Heart-Blood include palpitations, feelings of oppression and fullness in the chest, and chest pain. Cold hands, bluish lips and a slightly purple tongue are further indications of an impeded blood circulation. Although this condition creates signs and symptoms characterized by Fullness, it has arisen because of a failure of the Yang to transport and circulate blood.

That there is an underlying Ki- and Yang-deficient condition is made particularly apparent by the Ki-deficient condition of the Lungs. This pattern is manifesting in the patient through her breathlessness, tiredness, pallor and sweating during the day. This last symptom is a result of a weakness in the body's Defensive Ki (controlled by the Lungs) in regulating the pores of the skin. When Lung-Ki is weak the pores lose their tone and allow sweat to leak out spontaneously. Deficient Lung-Ki is further evident in the patient's Empty pulse and generally pale tongue.

It is clear that two patterns indicated here – that of stagnant Heart-Blood and Lung-Ki deficiency – are closely connected, and are both associated with a weakness of Gathering (or Chest) Ki. Gathering Ki provides both Organs with their motive force. Although the Heart Channel exhibits a Jitsu quality reflecting a degree of stasis, the underlying condition of the Organ is deficient. The Kyo Lung Channel more accurately reflects a basically deficient situation.

Treatment It is necessary in this instance to tonify the Ki and Yang of the Heart and Lungs without failing to assist the movement of Blood in the chest. Treatment should commence with an emphasis on tonifying Kyo, especially along the Lung Channel and in the chest. Tonification of the Tsubos Bladder-13, Directing Vessel-17 and Lung-9 will support this process. If the Heart Channel remains Jitsu in condition, gently disperse the Heart and possibly Heart Protector Channels (including Tsubos such as Heart Protector-6). This will help to regulate the flow of Blood in the chest.

(For details of treating Stagnation of Heart-Blood, see p.163, for Lung-Ki deficiency, see p.173.)

PART 4

Acupressure & Glossary of Tsubos
by Ilaira Bouratinos

This section describes how to find and use the most important tsubos[1] in your shiatsu practice. Stimulation of the tsubos with the intention of obtaining a specific result is a method that has been used for thousands of years in many traditional healing systems. There are numerous ancient and modern techniques that have been applied to the tsubos for the purpose of influencing the Ki of the channels and organs. The application of physical pressure (known as acupressure), the insertion of needles (known as acupuncture), the application of suction cups, magnets or special herbs and oils, are all traditional methods commonly employed in oriental bodywork systems.

Acupressure – the most direct and simple way to influence the Ki – offers shiatsu practitioners a unique tool for working on the body with great precision, while at the same time allowing them to employ the extensive range of shiatsu techniques used during a full body treatment. Many of the techniques can also be applied to oneself.

While routine stimulation of tsubos is achieved during a shiatsu treatment, there are cases where we may want to affect a specific body function or area which may not necessarily be directly related to the Zen Shiatsu diagnosis. Pressure applied to tsubos for their particular effects may therefore be given, either during, or independently of, the shiatsu treatment. Acupressure can therefore be viewed as a facet of, or adjunct to, Shiatsu and other systems of bodywork.

As you will see, the way the tsubos may be used can range from a modest 'prescription' of a single point, to choices based on complex and sophisticated analyses. Therefore, to avoid confusion, the key symptoms treated by each tsubo, are highlighted in *italics*. This does not mean that the other symptoms discussed are of less importance; it means only that those in italics are the ones most effectively treated by acupressure techniques. Certain adjuncts to treatment, such as the use of moxibustion and cupping[2], are also mentioned to encourage a broader scope of clinical applications.

Initially it is best to focus on understanding the main functions of the tsubos and acquire a thorough knowledge of the channel pathways, organ correspondences and special categories (classifications) into which tsubos are grouped (see Classification of Points on p.231). This knowledge will help you to understand how and why certain areas, tissues and body functions are influenced.

Shiatsu, as you already know, employs a wide variety of techniques, including stationary pressure, stretching, mobilisation and other methods such as rubbing or hacking (see chapters 3 and 5). Within this glossary, the term 'shiatsu' is used when the tsubo is effectively treated by a variety of bodywork techniques, as well as – or instead of – simple acupressure. Stretching, for example, may in some cases be the most effective method. Acupressure, by contrast, refers to those techniques applied directly to the tsubos, usually using the fingers or thumbs; although in some cases, stimulation of the tsubo can be achieved from a slightly wider area, with a variety of tools, including the palms, forearms, knees or feet.

HOW TO CHOOSE POINTS (TSUBOS)
Choosing a set of points that work together harmoniously to treat the whole person and the specific complaint, is accomplished according to the principles laid out over thousands of years of clinical experience by the doctors of the East. It is most important to remember that an effective choice of points

cannot be achieved without an accurate diagnosis. It is therefore of great importance to ensure the diagnosis is concise and clear.

In general, if the problems are primarily due to *deficiency and emptiness* or *kyo situations*, tsubos and techniques that bring the energy inwards, close to the centre of the body and to the affected area(s) are chosen. In this case tsubos on the affected area, or close to it, are of most significance. Such tsubos are known as *local points*.

Conversely, if there are many *jitsu manifestations* or symptoms of *excess and blockage* in the form of pathogenic factors or stagnation of Ki and Blood, tsubos and techniques that disperse, expel and move the Ki outwards, to the surface of the body and extremities are chosen. Therefore tsubos located far away from the problem, which are known as *distal points*, are of most importance.

Principles of point selection
Selection of points is directly related to the findings obtained from the diagnosis:

Selection of points according to the Channel Diagnosis
Appendix A,
The first level of diagnosis, collectively referred to as Channel Diagnosis, observes the channels, points and areas of the entire body as well as those directly related to the specific problem. This form of diagnosis is probably the most relevant aspect for bodywork practitioners, since continuous observation of the recipient's energy system occurs throughout the entire shiatsu session. In this context, Treatment is Diagnosis and Diagnosis is Treatment.

Selection of points will therefore initially be based on the findings obtained from the channel diagnosis. This is especially evident when dealing with problems of the channel pathways and pain conditions. A temporal headache, for example, may be treated according to the affected channels, the Gallbladder in this case.

Points are also selected to treat their Yin/Yang paired channel and organ, as well as the channel(s) related along the Six Divisions. Liv-3, may for example, be selected to treat the Gallbladder channel, whereas TH-5 may also be chosen in the same case, because the Triple Heater channel is related to the Gallbladder along the Six Divisions. Additionally other channels may also be affected at points of intersection (points where the channels cross over each other). A selection of local, adjacent and distal points should be combined.

Although Channel Diagnosis is always applicable in a shiatsu practice, there are cases where a more detailed differentiation is necessary.

Selection of points according to TCM Theory Diagnosis
Appendix B,
Differentiation of syndromes: Initially, the areas of the problem are located, and the main points that treat it are selected. Then, points that also treat the underlying disharmony of the person are chosen. A thorough evaluation of all the signs and symptoms and aspects of the person (physical, energetic, emotional, psychological, etc.) is necessary to reach an accurate diagnosis. This is achieved from the information obtained from the Four Methods of Diagnosis (see Part 3, p.189). The energetic analysis can be accomplished on various different levels, often with wide overlap areas. Contrary to Channel Diagnosis, internal diagnosis on one, or more of the six main levels of differentiation of syndromes is always applicable.

Firstly, a principle of treatment (treatment strategy) is formulated and points and techniques that tonify and nourish, or disperse excess are chosen from the Eight Principles Diagnosis. Points and techniques that influence the Ki, Blood, Body Fluids and Essence are chosen from the Vital Substances Diagnosis, whereas points and techniques that eliminate exterior or interior dampness, heat, fire, cold, phlegm, wind and dryness are chosen from the Pathogenic Factors (Six Evils) Diagnosis. Points of the affected channels are chosen according to their energetic quality and it's relationship to the disharmony determined by the Internal Organ Diagnosis.

An analysis of the patient's disharmony according to the Five Elements also offers a clear and precise method for selecting points. The Six Divisions differentiation offers a way to ensure that the chosen points have a direct influence on the affected channels and stage of development of the condition.

Selection of points from Empirical Knowledge and clinical practice
Appendix C,
This refers mainly to symptomatic treatments based on thousands of years of clinical experience by the doctors of the East and West.

CLASSIFICATION OF POINTS
All the body's points may be divided into two broad categories: those who's location and functions have been precisely charted and described, known as Fixed points or Classified points, and those that have not been charted, known as Transient points.

The first broad category includes all the Channel and Non-Channel points. The Channel points are grouped into various categories according to their energetic quality and the areas, substances and types of conditions they treat. The main categories of the points are discussed below. The Non-Channel points (also known as Extra, or Miscellaneous points) include both the traditional Extra points, mapped out thousands of years ago, and other more recently discovered ones. They are used in the treatment of specific conditions or body areas.

The second broad category, the Transient points, are points who's locations vary as they are a reflection of the particular disharmony and it's relationship to the person. They are therefore inherently unchartable. Transient points are found either as reactive points along the channel pathways and other specific areas worked during a Shiatsu treatment, or anywhere else on the body in which case they are known as Ashi points (meaning 'That's it'). Ashi points are found anywhere there is pain, tenderness or other abnormal sensation, manifesting either on palpation or spontaneously. They are usually used to treat pain conditions and their local area, but are also effective in other cases. Pain should be diminished after treatment.

SPECIAL POINT CATEGORIES (CLASSIFICATIONS)
The Bo and Yu points
Both the Yu and Bo points have an immediate and powerful effect on their pertaining organs. They may be tender either spontaneously or on palpation and are therefore also useful in diagnosis. The use of Bo and Yu points together constitute a particularly powerful treatment.

The Bo points, also known as Alarm or Front Collecting points, are located on the chest and abdomen, directly above their pertaining organs (see Fig 18.6 on page 208). It is here that the Ki of each of the internal organs converges and accumulates. The Bo points have an immediate and direct effect on the internal organs and are used more often in acute conditions to treat the Yang Organs. The Bo points are:

Lung	Lu-1	Heart	Ren-14	Heart Protector	Ren-17
Large Intestine	St-25	Small Intestine	Ren-4	Triple Heater	Ren-5
Stomach	Ren-12	Bladder	Ren-3	Gall Bladder	GB-24
Spleen	Liv-13	Kidney	GB-25	Liver	Liv-14

The Yu points, also known as Associated or Back Transporting points, are located on the back directly above their pertaining organs to which they send, or 'transport' Ki directly (see fig 18.5 on page 207). They have a direct tonifying influence on the internal organs and are used in both acute and chronic conditions, especially when there is depletion of the vital substances. The Yu points also treat the orifices that pertain to their associated organ. The Yu points are:

Lung	Bl-13	Heart	Bl-15	Heart Protector	Bl-14
Large Intestine	Bl-25	Small Intestine	Bl-27	Triple Heater	Bl-22
Stomach	Bl-21	Bladder	Bl-28	Gall Bladder	Bl-19
Spleen	Bl-20	Kidney	Bl-23	Liver	Bl-18

Additional Yu points (not directly related to the Zangfu organs)

Governing Vessel	BI-16	Sea of Ki	BI-24	Backbone (lower spine)	BI-29
Diaphragm (and Blood)	BI-17	Original Ki Gate	BI-26	Anus	BI-30

The Source Points

The Source point for each of the twelve regular channels are found at the wrists and ankles. They have a profound tonifying effect on the underlying energy of the organs and are very important in the treatment of any chronic condition, particularly when there is depletion of the vital substances. This is because the Original (Source) Ki emerges here. They are of most significance on the Yin channels. The Source points are: **Lu-9, LI-4, St-42, Sp-3, He-7, SI-4, Bl-64, Kd-3, HP-7, TH-4, GB-40** and **Liv-3**.

The Accumulation Points

Also known as Cleft points, these are where the Ki of the channels accumulates, just as water gathers in a crevice or cleft. They are therefore used to treat acute, excess conditions either of the organ itself or the channel, particularly when there is pain. On the Yin channels they also treat disorders of the Blood (including heat and stasis of Blood). The Accumulation points are: **Lu-6, LI-7, St-34, Sp-8, He-6, SI-6, Bl-63, Kd-5, HP-4, TH-7, GB-36** and **Liv-6**.

The Connecting Points

The Connecting points offer a connection via the Yin-Yang related channels. They are therefore used to harmonise the Ki of the paired channels and organs. They are often used to 'transfer' an excess pathogen from one organ to another (usually from the Yin channel to it's Yang pair). Connecting points are also useful in the treatment of channel disorders and emotional problems. The Connecting points are: **Lu-7, LI-6, St-40, Sp-4, He-5, SI-7, Bl-58, Kd-4, HP-6, TH-5, GB-37** and **Liv-5**. There are also three additional connecting points: Sp-21, the Great Connecting point of the Spleen, DU-1 Connecting point for the Governing Vessel, and REN-15 for the Directing Vessel.

The Six Command Points

These points have a special influence on, and are used to treat problems of, a particular body area.

Abdomen	St-36	Thorax/Chest	HP-6	Face and Mouth	LI-4
Back	BI-40	Head and back of neck	Lu-7	Consciousness	Du-26

The Eight Gathering Points

Also called Influential or Meeting points, these are points where the energy of the organs, certain tissues and vital substances gathers and accumulates. The Gathering points have a direct influence on these and are used to treat various conditions affecting them.

Ki	Ren-17	Yin Organs	Liv-13	Bones	BI-11
Sinews	GB-34	Blood	BI-17	Yang Organs	Ren-12
Marrow	GB-39	Blood Vessels	Lu-9		

The Five Transporting Points

The Five Transporting points are five points on each channel, located distal to the elbows and knees, whose quality of Ki is likened to the flow of water along it's course, starting at a well and reaching a distant ocean. Each of these points has an individual energetic character that distinguishes the nature of the Ki flowing through it. This is irrespective of the other categories they are grouped into. The Five Transporting points can also be classified in relation to the Five Elements; meaning that they are also employed in the treatment of imbalances between the Elements. The Five Element points correspond to the Five Transporting points:

		Well point	Spring point	Stream point	River point	Sea point
Yin channel	controls	Wood → produces Fire	→ Earth	→ Metal	→ Water	
Yang channel		Metal → Water	→ Wood	→ Fire	→ Earth	

The Well Points

These are located at the distal ends of the Twelve Regular channels, at the tips of the fingers and toes. At these points, the Ki of the channels is at it's most superficial, flowing rapidly in an outward direction. It is here that the polarity of Yin/Yang changes as the paired channels flow into one another. The well points have a powerful calming effect on the mind and are used for insomnia, anxiety, irritability and to restore consciousness. They also activate the channel pathways in cases of pain and other channel disorders. On the Yin channels they pertain to the Wood Element, and on the Yang, to the Metal Element.

The Spring points

The second points along the channels, they are located at the base of the fingers and toes. The Ki here is likened to the water in a swirling spring, being similar to that of the well points insofar as it is dynamic and moves rapidly. These points are used to clear pathogenic factors, particularly heat and fire. On the Yin channels they pertain to Fire, and on the Yang, to Water.

The Stream points

The third points along the channels, these are located on the wrists and ankles on the Yin channels and on the metacarpals and metatarsals on the Yang channels. The Ki here, although still moving quickly, begins to enter a little deeper into the circulation and becomes wider. It is at these points that pathogens penetrate deeper into the channels, and the Defensive Ki gathers here to protect the interior of the body. On the Yin channels they are primarily used to tonify and nourish the organs, and on the Yang, to expel pathogenic factors. On the Yin channels they are also Source points and belong to the Earth Element. On the Yang channels they belong to Wood.

Yin channel points	Well Wood	Spring Fire	Stream Earth	River Metal	Sea Water
Lung	11	10	9	8	5
Spleen	1	2	3	5	9
Heart	9	8	7	4	3
Kidney	1	2	3	7	10
Heart Protector	9	8	7	5	3
Liver	1	2	3	4	8
Yang channel points	**Well** Metal	**Spring** Water	**Stream** Wood	**River** Fire	**Sea** Earth
Large Intestine	1	2	3	5	11
Stomach	45	44	43	41	36
Small Intestine	1	2	3	5	8
Bladder	67	66	65	60	40
Triple Heater	1	2	3	6	10
Gall Bladder	44	43	41	38	34

The River points

They are located on the forearm and leg on the Yin channels and pertain to Metal, whereas on the Yang channels they are found at the wrists and ankles and pertain to Fire. The Ki at the River points flows like a strong current after coming a long distance from its source. The Ki at these points is much bigger, wider and deeper and it is here that pathogens enter into the joints, tendons and bones. River points are commonly used in the treatment of painful obstruction syndrome and arthritis.

The Sea points

Located at the elbows and knees, they are where the Ki of the channel becomes deep and joins the systemic circulation of the body, like a river flowing into the sea. The Ki at these points moves slowly inwards towards the pertaining organ. The Sea points have a deeper but less immediate effect. They are used to harmonise the Ki of the internal organs in both acute and chronic conditions by clearing interior pathogenic factors and regulating the flow of Ki. They also tonify the vital substances. On the Yin channels they belong to the Water Element, and on the Yang channels, to the Earth Element. There are three additional sea points, known as the *Lower sea points*, one each for the Large Intestine, Small Intestine and Triple Heater. They are **St-37**, **St-39** and **Bl-39** respectively.

Selecting points according to the Five Elements

In cases of deficiency of an Element the point pertaining to the 'Mother Element' is chosen to tonify it. For example, in the case of deficiency of the Wood Element, the point Liv-8 is chosen (Liver pertains to Wood and Liv-8 is a Water point: Water generates [produces] Wood). These points are known as
  Tonification points and are: **Lu-9**, **LI-11**, **St-41**, **Sp-2**, **He-9**, **SI-3**, **Bl-67**, **Kd-7**, **HP-9**, **TH-3**, **GB-43** and **Liv-8**.

In the case of excess the 'Child Element' point is dispersed (sedated) – for example Liver fire may be treated using the point Liv-2 (Liv-2 is a fire point: Fire is the child of Wood and therefore sedates it). The
  Sedation points are: **Lu-5**, **LI-2**, **St-45**, **Sp-5**, **He-7**, **SI-8**, **Bl-65**, **Kd-1**, **HP-7**, **TH-10**, **GB-38** and **Liv-2**.

Another, less widespread use of the Five Element points is the reinforcing of a particular element using the **Horary points:** these points belong to the same Element as the one we want to affect. For example we could use Lu-8 to reinforce the Lung Ki (Lu-8 is a Metal point and the Lungs pertain to Metal). The
  Horary points are **Lu-8**, **LI-1**, **St-36**, **Sp-3**, **He-8**, **SI-5**, **Bl-66**, **Kd-10**, **HP-8**, **TH-6**, **GB-41** and **Liv-1**.

The Five Element points are also employed in the treatment of emotional disorders or conditions associated with the pathogenic factors. In the latter case Water points treat cold, dampness and phlegm conditions, Wood points treat wind, Fire points treat heat and fire, Earth points treat dampness and phlegm, and Metal points treat dryness.

The Five Element method of points' selection is generally combined with the other actions a point may have. One must look at all the energetic qualities of a point in order to make the most effective choice. He-9, for example, is the Tonification point for the Heart, but is not as often used to treat deficiency of the Heart as He-7 because well points are mostly used in the treatment of acute conditions.

THE EIGHT EXTRAORDINARY VESSELS

The Eight Extraordinary Vessels, unlike the Twelve Regular channels, are not directly related to individual Zangfu organs, although they do have a close relationship to the Kidneys, uterus and brain. They aid the flow of Ki and Blood in the regular channels by acting as reservoirs (the Twelve Primary Channels are more like rivers). When there is a surplus of Ki and Blood in the regular channels it overflows into the Extraordinary Vessels. Conversely the Ki and Blood from the Extraordinary Vessels are transferred to the Regular Channels as needed. The latter may occur in times of greater demand such as during a chronic illness, shock or pregnancy. 'The Eight Extraordinary Vessels are so named because they do not conform to the norm. Ki and Blood constantly flow through the twelve regular channels and, when abundant, overflow into the Extraordinary Vessels.'[3]

This emptying and filling of the Extraordinary Vessels ensures there is always a constant and uninterrupted flow of Ki and Blood in the regular Channels in order that that homeostasis may be maintained to the maximum. Thus the Extraordinary Vessels do not have their own continuous pattern of circulation but rather respond to the fluctuations of the twelve major channels. One classical text says 'When there are heavy rains, canals and ditches are full to the brim … similarly, the extraordinary vessels are left out of the channel system so that they can take the overflow from the main channels'.[4]

The Extraordinary Vessels regulate the circulation of Essence acting as a link between the Pre-Heaven and Post-Heaven Ki. They are mostly used to treat problems of the Essence and constitution. The Penetrating and Conception Vessels particularly influence the cycles of the Essence that control growth, development, reproduction and the ageing process. Each cycle lasts seven years in women and eight years in men.

The Penetrating, Conception and Governing Vessels also circulate the Defensive Ki over the thorax, abdomen and back thus aiding in the protection of the body from exterior pathogenic factors.[5]

The Opening and Coupled points for the Eight Extraordinary Vessels

With the exception of the Directing and Governing Vessels, the Extraordinary Vessels do not have their own points but rather share the points of the Twelve Regular Channels. Their Ki is accessed via a special point that 'opens' it, known as the **Opening point** (also called the Master point) and a paired point to the opening point known as the **Coupled point**. These are listed below. The Extraordinary Vessels may be grouped into pairs according to their Yin/Yang polarity. Their Opening and Coupled points are listed below:

Governing Vessel	*Opening point* SI-3	*Coupled point* Bl-62
Yang Heel Vessel	*Opening point* Bl-62	*Coupled point* SI-3
Directing Vessel	*Opening point* Lu-7	*Coupled point* Kd-6
Yin Heel Vessel	*Opening point* Kd-6	*Coupled point* Lu-7
Penetrating Vessel	*Opening point* Sp-4	*Coupled point* HP-6
Yin Linking Vessel	*Opening point* HP-6	*Coupled point* Sp-4
Girdle Vessel	*Opening point* GB-41	*Coupled point* TH-5
Yang Linking Vessel	*Opening point* TH-5	*Coupled point* GB-41

The **Governing Vessel** runs along the posterior midline ascending to the head and face and joining all the Yang Meridians at DU-14. It is considered to be the most Yang of all the channels and is known as the 'Sea of Yang'.

The **Directing Vessel** (also called **Conception Vessel**) ascends across the abdomen and chest, reaching the face. It connects all the Yin meridians and is known as the 'Sea of Yin'.

The **Penetrating Vessel**, also known as the 'Sea of Blood', runs parallel to the Kidney channel up the legs, through the abdomen and chest to the face. It connects the twelve regular channels and acts as a reservoir for their Ki and Blood.

The **Yin Linking Vessel** connects and regulates the flow of Ki in all the Yin channels and dominates the interior of the body.

The **Yin Heel Vessel** starts on the medial aspect of the heel and travels up the inside of the body with the Kidney channel to the face where it joins the Yang Heel Vessel at the inner canthus. It regulates the ascending and descending of Yin Ki.

The **Yang Heel Vessel** starts on the lateral aspect of the heel and travels up the lateral sides of the body to join the Yin Heel meridian at the eyes. It regulates the ascending and descending of Yang Ki and movement of the lower limbs.

The **Yang Linking Vessel** connects and regulates the flow of Ki in all the Yang channels and dominates the exterior of the body.

The **Girdle Vessel** (also known as the 'belt meridian') originates at the hypochondrium, encircles the waist and binds all the other channels.

THE SIX DIVISIONS

There are Twelve Regular Channels divided into six Yin channels and six Yang channels. These channels are grouped into two sets of six pairs.

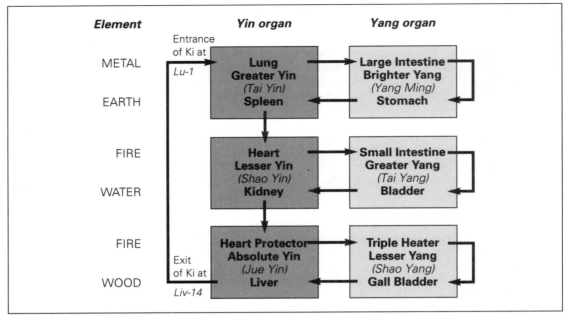

The Six Divisions.

The first set is known as the *interiorly/exteriorly related channels,* or simply the *Yin/Yang paired channels.* These pairs consist of the Yin and Yang channel belonging to the same Element; they are: Lung – Large Intestine; Spleen – Stomach; Heart – Small Intestine; Heart Protector – Triple Heater; Liver – Gallbladder; Kidney – Bladder. The Yin/Yang paired channels meet at the tips of the fingers and toes, where the polarity of Yin/Yang changes.

The Twelve Regular Channels are further subdivided into three pairs of Yin and three pairs of Yang channels known as the *Six Divisions.* The three pairs of Yang channels related along the Six Divisions meet at the face whereas the Yin channels meet on the chest.

Schematic representation of the channel distribution on the four limbs.

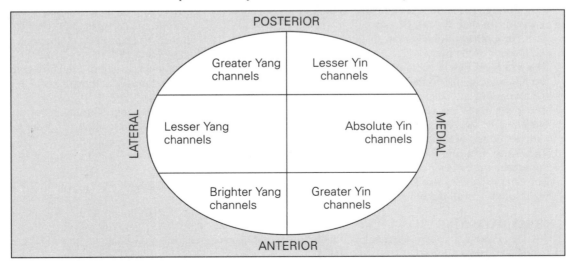

The Six Divisions reflect a similarity of the energy flowing in the upper and lower limbs.

The channels running along the antero-medial surface of the limbs are known as the **Greater Yin channels**. Those running along the antero-lateral surface of the limbs are known as the **Brighter Yang channels**. Those running along the middle of the medial surface of the limbs are known as the **Absolute Yin channels**. Those running along the middle of the lateral surface of the limbs are known as the **Lesser Yang channels**. Those running along the postero-medial surface of the limbs are known as the **Lesser Yin Channels** and finally those running along the postero-lateral surface of the limbs are known as the **Greater Yang channels**.

The Six Divisions are also used in diagnosis to ascertain the depth of a disease and it's progression from the exterior to the interior of the body or vice versa.

THE CHINESE CLOCK

As the rhythms of nature fluctuate from day to night, winter to summer and so on, so the Ki in the channels waxes and wanes. There are numerous cycles the Ki follows from day to day, year to year, spanning the whole of our lifetime.

During the daily 24 hour cycle, the Ki surges through each of the 12 channels for two hours. It does this following the Six Divisions schema: starting at 3am the Ki enters the Lung channel and every two hours flows to the next, ending at the Liver.

Thus each channel has a particular time of day when it contains a particularly large supply of Ki and an opposite time of day when it's Ki level is at it's lowest. This is useful information because it indicates that a symptom occurring daily at the same time *may* be related to the channel which has its peak of Ki is at that time, or the one that has it's lowest level of Ki. A problem occurring around 5 a.m. may therefore be related to either the Large Intestine or the Kidney, or to both.

The Chinese Clock.

POINT LOCATION AND APPLICATION OF PRESSURE

The points may be seen as doorways or windows that when 'opened' cause a channel or area of the body to be activated, in a similar way to a door opening into a passageway of a building. Therefore when the points are properly stimulated a 'Ki sensation' should always be achieved. This sensation, called '*De Qi*' in Chinese (meaning: to find the Ki [of the point]) indicates that the Ki has been accessed, i.e. the 'door' has been opened and the 'breeze' can clearly be felt.

This sensation varies from person to person and is different from one channel or point to another. Moreover, it depends on the nature and location of the imbalance and the constitutional energy of the person. The *de qi* sensation has been described by thousands of people throughout the centuries with terms such as: a relieving ache or pain, a spreading out sensation (to the affected areas), a distending soreness, a warm feeling, a tingling or numbness, a distending or even electric sensation. When the *de qi* sensation 'arrives' we can be sure we have accessed the point properly.

If there is no sensation at all one of the following has occurred: (a) the pressure was not applied in the right location (i.e. the point was mis-located) (b) the pressure was not applied correctly (either at the wrong angle, too superficially or without Ki projection) or (c) the person is extremely deficient in Ki and Blood.

When the term *pain* is used by your client, two questions should be asked: (a) does the pain feel like something is being bruised or injured? or (b) is there also a sensation of 'release' or something opening up at the same time? The first type of pain may be considered as a *Bad Pain* and indicates wrongly applied pressure. This may be due to any of the following: the pressure was applied at the wrong angle or location, was applied too suddenly or too strongly, or was applied without Ki projection. The second type of pain may be considered as a *Good Pain* (as long at is not too excessive) and indicates that stuck Ki is being released.

A note on Cun

Cun (body inches) are relative to the body area to which they pertain. For example 1" on the abdomen may be a slightly different size to 1" on the forearm or face.

General guidelines

1" is approximately the length of the middle phalanx of the middle finger, or slightly more than one thumb's width.

3" is approximately the width of the four fingers at the level of the first interphalangeal joint of the index finger.

Cun measurements according to body area

Head, face and neck

• Anterior to posterior hairline	–12"
• Between eyebrows (Yin Tang) to anterior hairline	–3"
• Yin Tang to posterior hairline	–15"
• DU-14 to posterior hairline	–3"
• St-8 to St-8 (or left to right mastoid processes)	–9"
• Eye, inner to outer canthus	–1"

Chest, back and abdomen

• Centre of axilla to just below the floating ribs	–12"
• Anterior midline to acromion	–8"
• Anterior midline to midmammilary line	–4"
• Umbilicus to xiphisternal junction	–8"
• Anterior midline to lateral border of the rectus Abdominis muscle or medial aspect of ASIS	–4"
• Umbilicus to upper border of pubic symphysis	–5"
• Posterior midline to medial border of scapula	–3"
• Medial border of PSIS to posterior midline	–1.5"

Upper Limb
- Upper arm, anterior axillary fold to cubital crease   –9"
- Forearm, cubital to wrist crease (or LI-5 to LI-11)   –12"

Lower Limb
- Upper border of greater trochanter to knee crease   –19"
- Protruberance of greater trochanter to knee crease   –18"
- Gluteal crease to popliteal crease   –14"
- Patella: superior to inferior borders   –2"
- Medial malleolus to knee crease-inner eye the knee   –15"
- Lateral malleolus to knee crease (or St-35)   –16"

To supplement the location of the points according to cun measurement, many of the points listed have additional guidelines for location in order to guide the Shiatsu practitioner to the right area – to then find the point using Ki sensitivity. This is actually of far more importance than the cun measurements ("), which are mentioned mainly for reference. Many points can be affected by a wider area from a Shiatsu point of view, than by the acupuncturist's pin-point and should always be located where they are felt to be most reactive.

Useful anatomical landmarks for point location
- Medial angle of scapula (root of scapula spine)   -level with T3
- Inferior angle of scapula   -level with T7
- Free end of 12th rib   -level with L2
- Top of iliac crest   -level with L4
- Dimple of Venues   -level with the lower border of L5
- High point of PSIS   -level with second sacral foramen

CAUTIONS AND CONTRAINDICATIONS
There are cases where certain points should be used with great care or not at all, referred to throughout this text as *cautioned* and *contraindicated points* respectively. To avoid unsuitable treatment that may result in depletion or 'confusion' of the Ki, always ensure that the diagnosis, principle of treatment and choice of points are appropriate.

General Cautions
Avoid overstimulation or excessive pressure on weak, elderly or over-deficient patients, during pregnancy, and in patients whose Ki and Blood is very empty.

Contraindications
Points that descend the Ki or move the Ki strongly in the uterus and lower burner should be avoided altogether during pregnancy, on women with heavy menstrual flow and in other situations where the Ki of the lower burner must be raised upwards rather than descended (e.g. dizziness, exhaustion, frequent urination and prolapses due to sinking of the Ki). Pressure applied directly downwards on the points of the thorax and top of shoulder (particularly GB-21) will cause the Ki to descend and should therefore be avoided when the conditions described above are present. Stimulation to LI-4, Sp-6 and other surrounding points of the inner calf should also be avoided in these situations, and points of the lower back and abdomen should be treated with caution. Bl-60 and Bl-67 are also contraindicated during pregnancy.

Great care should be taken when working on the neck so as to avoid overstimulation or over stretching the area. This is particularly important in elderly or very weak patients and those suffering from arthritis or osteoporosis of the spine and hypertension.

APPENDIX A
POINTS ACCORDING TO AREA

Diseased area	Local Points	Distal Points
Head		
whole head	Du-20	Liv-3, Kd-1, Kd-6
vertex	Du-20, Du-23	Liv-3, Kd-1
temple	Tai Yang, GB-8, GB-20	TH-5, GB-41
forehead	St-8, Du-23, GB-14, Yin Tang	LI-4, St-41, St-44
occiput and neck	Bl-10, Du-14, Du-16	SI-3, Lu-7, GB-39, SI-6, Bl-60, -67
Face		
face	varying	LI-4, St-44, Lu-7, TH-5
eyes	Bl-1, Bl-2, GB-1, St-1, St-2, TH-23, Tai Yang, St-3	Liv-3, GB-37, GB-20, LI-4, Kd-6, Liv-2, -3
nose	LI-19, LI-20, Du-23, Yin Tang, Bi Tong	Lu-7, LI-4
teeth	St-6, St-4, Ren-24	LI-4, St-44, Lu-7
ears	TH-21, SI-19, GB-2, TH-16, -17, GB-20	TH-3, -5, GB-41, GB-43, GB-39, Kd-3, -6
tongue	Ren-23	He-5, Du-15, Kd-6
throat	St-9, LI-18, SI-17, Ren-23	Lu-10, Lu-11, Kd-6
neck	Du-14, -15, -16, Bai Lao, Bl-10, -11, Huatuo points, SI-13, -14, -15	SI-3, Lu-7, GB-39 LI-4, Liv-2, LI-1, Lu-7, Luozhen
Trunk		
chest	Ren-17, Lu-1, Liv-14, Kd-25, St-12-18, Bl-13-18, Sp-20, -21	HP-6, Lu-5, LI-4, St-40, Sp-4
breasts	Ren-17, St-18, Liv-14, HP-1	HP-6, GB-41, Sp- 4, SI-1
Abdomen		
abdomen	Ren-4, Ren-6	St-36
epigastrium	Ren-12, St-21, Bl-21, Liv-14	St-36, Sp-4, HP-6
middle of abdomen	St-25, Sp-15, Ren-8, Bl-25, Bl-27	St-36, St-37, St-39
lower abdomen	Ren-3, -4, -5, -6, Bl-23, Bl-25	Sp-6, Sp-8, Sp-9, St-36, Bl-40
bladder	Ren-3, St-28, Bl-28	Sp-6 & 9
genitals	Ren-2, -3, -4, St-29, -30, Zigong	Sp-6, -9, Liv-5, GB-41, Kd-5, Bl-67
sides of abdomen	Liv-13, -14, GB-24, -27, -28, Bl-18, -19	TH-6, GB-34, GB-41, Liv-3
Lumbar region		
lumbar region	Bl-23, -25, -52, Du-4, 17th vertebra pt., Huatuo points	Bl-40, -60, GB-30, Du-26, Yaotong, Du-26, YinTang, LI-4, He-7
rectum	Bl-30, Du-1	Bl-57
Upper limb		
upper limb	varying, LI-10	Huatuo points C5-T1
shoulder	TH-14, LI-15, GB-21	St-38, TH-5, LI- 4 & 11, TH-5
elbow	LI-10, 11, 12, SI-8, TH-10, Lu-5	LI-4, TH-5, SI-6, GB-34
wrist	TH-4, 5, LI- 5, SI-4, HP-7, Lu-9	GB-40
Lower limb		
lower limb	varying, St-36	Huatuo points L3-S1
hip	GB-29, GB-30, St-31	GB-34, GB-41
knee	St-35 & 36, Sp- 9, Bl-39 & 40	Bl-23
ankle	Bl-60 & 62, Kd-6, St-41, GB-40	TH-4

APPENDIX B
DIFFERENTIATION OF SYNDROMES AND POINTS

Points chosen from the Eight Principles, Vital Substances and Pathogenic Factors diagnosis

Ki

Ki deficiency	St-36, Ren-6, Lu-9, Sp-3, Ren-12, -17, Bl-20, 21
Ki Stagnation	GB-34, Liv-3, -14, TH-5
Sinking Ki	Du-20, St-36

Blood

Blood deficiency	Sp-6, Ren-4, St-36, Liv-8, Bl-15, -17, -20, -21, -23, Liv-3, He-7, Sp-10
Blood heat	He-8, HP-8, Liv-2, -3, Sp-10, Bl-40, LI-11
Blood stasis	Liv-3, Sp-4, -6, -8, -10, HP-6, Ren-17, Bl-17, -18
Blood loss	Sp-1, -10, Bl-17, Liv-1, -14

Body Fluids

Dampness	Sp-3, -9, -6, Bl-20, -22, -23, Ren-4, -6, Liv-13.
Phlegm	St-40, Sp-3, Lu-5, Bl-20, -13
Oedema	Kd-3, -7, Sp-6, -9, Lu-7, LI-4, Bl-22, -23, Ren-9
Dryness	Ren-12, St-36, Kd-6, Lu-7, Sp-6, Kd-7

Essence

Decline of the Kidney Essence	Du-4, Bl-23, -52, Kd-3, Sp-6, GB-39, Du-16, Bl-11, Ren-4

Shen

Restlessness of the mind	He-7, -5, SI-3, HP-6, -7, Sp-6, Kd-1, -6, Bl-15, -43, -44, LI-4, Liv-3
Loss of consciousness	Du-26, the twelve well points

Yin Yang

Yin deficiency	Kd-6, Sp-6, Lu-7, Ren-4, -12, Bl-23
Yang deficiency	St-36, Kd-3, Ren-6, Bl-23, Ren-20
Yin collapse	Kd-3, -7, Ren-6, -4
Yang collapse	Ren-8, St-36, Kd-3, Du-20, Ren-6, -12

Other Pathogenic factors

Exterior cold	Lu-7, LI-4, Bl-12, -13
Interior cold	St-36, Sp-6, Kd-3, Ren-4, -6, -8, -12, Du-4
Exterior wind	Lu-7, LI-4, TH-5, Bl-12, -13, Du-14, -15, Bl-10
Interior wind	Liv-1, -3, Bl-18, Du-16, GB-20, Du-20 and the other Well points.
Fire	Liv-2, St-44, He-8, HP-8, Lu-10, LI-4, -11, Liv-3, Kd-1, Du-14

APPENDIX C
SYMPTOMS AND POINTS

Symptoms	Points
Abdominal distension and pain	St-36, -37, Sp-4, -6, -3, Ren-4, -6, St-25, Ren-12, LI-4, -11
Asthma	Ren-22, -17, Ding Chuan, LI-4
Breast swelling and pain	Liv-14, St-18, Liv-3, GB-41, HP-1, -6, St-36
Chest pain	Ren-17, HP-4, -6, LI-4
Cough	Lu-1, -7, Bl-12, -13, LI-4
Cough with profuse phlegm	Lu-1, -5, St-40
Cough, unproductive, dry	Lu-9, -7, Kd-6, St-36
Coma or fainting	Du-26, the twelve well points, Kd-1
Constipation	Sp-15, St-25, Bl-25, Ren-6, -4, Sp-6, TH-6, LI-4, St-37
Cystitis	Ren-3, St-28, Bl-23, -28, Sp-6, -9, Liv-5, -8
Diarrhoea	St-25, Sp-9, St-36, -37, Ren-8 (moxa)
Dysmenorrhoea	Sp-4, -6, Liv-3, Ren-4, St-25, GB-27, -28, Bl-23, -32
Epigastric pain	Ren-12, HP-6, St-34, -36, Bl-21
Fainting, loss of consciousness	Du-26, -20, Ren-4, St-36, LI-4, HP-9, Kd-1
Fullness of the chest	HP-6, Ren-17, Lu-1, LI-4, Lu-7
Fever	Du-14, LI-4, -11, Lu-10, Liv-3
Genital pain or itching	Liv-5, Sp-6, St-30, Bl-32
Haemorrhage	Sp-1, -10 (moxa)
Haemorrhoids	Du-1, -20, Bl-57, Sp-6, Bl-30
Hiccup (spasm of the diaphragm)	HP-6, St-12, -13, St-20, GB-24, Liv-14, Bl-17, St-36
Hypertension	St-9, Liv-2, -3, LI-11, -4, Sp-6, Kd-6, GB-20
Hypochondrial pain	GB-34, TH-6, HP-6, TH-5, Liv-14, GB-41, Bl-17, -18, -19, -20
Indigestion	St-36, Sp- 4, Ren-12, St-25, HP-6
Infertility	Bl-23, -52, Sp-4, -6, Kd-3, Ren-4, -6, St-30, -36
Impotence, premature ejaculation	Ren-4, Sp- 6, Kd-3, Bl-23, -52, St-30, Kd-3
Insomnia	He-7, Sp-6, Kd-6, GB-13, Anmian
Insufficient lactation	SI-1, St-18, -36, Ren-17
Labour (delayed or prolonged)	Bl-31, -32, Sp-6, Liv-3, -5, LI-4, GB-21, Bl-60, -67
Malposition of the foetus	Bl-67 (moxa)
Mastitis	Liv-14, St-18, Ren-17, Liv-2, SI-1, HP-6
Miscarriage, threatened	Sp-1, Du-20, St-36, -30
Morning sickness in pregnancy	Ren-12, HP-6, St-36, -30, Bl-20, -21
Nausea and vomiting	HP-6, St-21, -36
Pain, anywhere	LI-4, Liv-3, Sp-21, Bl-17, TH-5, HP-6, GB-34, Du-26
Palpitations	H-7, HP-4, -6, Ren-17, Bl-15
Poor appetite	St-36, Sp-3, Ren-12, Bl-20, -21
Prolapse of the uterus or rectum	Du-20, St-36, -30, Du-1, Bl-30, -32
Salivation, excessive	Ren-24, Du-26, St-4, -6, LI-4, Sp-3, LI-4
Sciatica	Bl-23, -30, GB-30, -34, Bl-36, GB-31, Bl-40, -57, -60
Sore throat	LI-4, Lu-10, -11, LI-1, -18, St-9, Lu-1
Sweating excessive	LI-4, Kd-7, Du-14, Liv-3, LI-11, He-6
Sweating, spontaneous	LI-4, Kd-7, St-36, Lu-9, -7, Du-14, Bai Lao
Sweating, night	He-6, Kd-7, SI-3, LI-4, Bl-43, Du-14
Sweating, absence	LI-4, Lu-7, Bl-13, Kd-7, SI-3
Temporomandibular syndrome	St-6, -7, LI-4, GB-34, TB-5
Vaginal discharge (leucorrhoea)	GB-26, Sp-6, Ren-6, Sp-9, St-36, Kd-3, GB-41
Weakness, general	St-36, Ren-4, -6, Du-4, Bl-23, Liv-13
Weakness of the limbs	St-36, Liv-13, Sp-3, LI-10

Glossary of Tsubos

THE LUNG CHANNEL
Greater Yin channel of the upper limb

Lung-1

On the lateral aspect of the chest, 6" lateral to the anterior midline. Inferior and slightly lateral to Lu-2, level with the first intercostal space, on the pectoralis major muscle. To aid location stretch the patient's arm out forward (flexion of the shoulder).

Applications

Lu-1, the Bo point for the Lungs, has a powerful effect on the entire thorax, chest, and respiratory system by promoting the Lung dispersing and descending functions. It therefore clears, relaxes and disperses fullness from the chest, stops pain and descends rebellious Ki from the Upper and Middle Burners. Lu-1 is one of the main points to treat *cough, asthma with dyspnoea*, fullness, oppression and *pain of the chest*, particularly if *worse when lying down*. It is used in conditions such as: bronchitis, pain and swelling of the throat, blocked nose and fever due to interior heat in the Lungs, chills and fever due to exterior pathogenic factors, exhaustion with difficulty lying down, nausea and vomiting brought on by coughing, pain of the shoulder and upper back. Lu-1 is 'the entrance point of Ki' (i.e.first point in the cycle of Ki) [whereas Liv-14 is the last]. It may therefore also be used to tonify and stimulate the Ki of the entire body, ease stagnation of Ki in the chest and abdomen and smooth the Liver. Combine Lu-1 with Bl-13 to treat acute or chronic cough due to either excess or deficiency, or with St-40 and Lu-5 for cough due to phlegm and heat in the Lungs, or with HP-6, LI-4, Liv-3 and Ren-17 for chest pain.

Treatment

Pressure is applied down and inwards to the chest. Dispersing stimulation may be used superficially to treat exterior problems whereas stronger pressure is used to disperse interior stagnation. A distending sensation should be felt radiating down into the chest and lungs to the diaphragm and reaching the abdomen, or spreading out across the front of the chest and shoulder to the arm, extending to the upper back, neck, throat or face. Shiatsu is best applied in a supine position (with the arm down by side at an angle of approximately 45°) or in a sitting position with the arm stretched out forward. **Caution:** Avoid excessive pressure to Lu-1 (and other points of the thorax) in patients suffering from heart disease. Over stimulation may in some cases aggravate the respiratory system causing an asthma attack (in predisposed patients). Do not to overstimulate the Lung descending functions during pregnancy, heavy menstrual bleeding and in very deficient patients.

Lung-2

In the large depression of the infraclavicular fossa, between the deltoid and pectoralis major muscles, in the delto-pectoral triangle. It is medial to the coracoid process of the scapula, approximately 6" lateral to the anterior midline. To aid it's location flex the patient's shoulder.

Applications and treatment
Similar to Lu-1. It is particularly effective in treating shoulder problems with *difficulty in adduction* (e.g. frozen shoulder). It is not as commonly used as Lu-1 for interior Lung conditions.

Lung-5
On the cubital crease, in the deep depression on the radial side of the tendon of the biceps brachii muscle (medial to the brachioradialis muscle). Locate with the elbow slightly flexed.

Applications
Lu-5 clears both full and empty heat from the Lungs, resolves phlegm, descends rebellious Lung Ki and strengthens Lung Yin. It is commonly used to treat *chronic productive phlegm* and/or *Lung heat conditions* such as *bronchitis*, pneumonia and *asthma* manifesting with symptoms including: *productive cough, thick yellow, dark, turbid sputum, dry cough*, coughing blood, fever, *dyspnoea, shortness of breath*, dry throat, pain, *fullness and heaviness of the chest*. It is also used to treat vomiting, frequent urination, enuresis, oedema, diarrhoea, swelling of the four limbs, pain of the elbow and arm. Combine Lu-5 with St-40 and Sp-3 for very productive cough due to damp phlegm in the Lungs, or with Lu-7 and LI-4 for asthma and with LI-11 for tennis elbow.

Treatment
Shiatsu is best applied in a supine position with the forearm supinated and the elbow either extended or flexed. A sensation should radiate deep into the cubital fossa and up the arm to the shoulder and chest or down the forearm toward the wrist.

Lung-6
Along the line drawn from Lu-5 to Lu-9, 7" above Lu-9 (5" below Lu-5), on the brachioradialis muscle.

Applications
Clears excess conditions from the Lung, particularly heat, stops pain and bleeding. Common symptoms it is used for include: *nosebleed* and coughing blood; loss of voice; fever without sweating; cough and sore throat due to interior full heat in the Lung; acute asthma attack; pain of the forearm, elbow and arm, and impaired flexion of the elbow.

Treatment
Acupressure is best applied in a supine or sitting position. A sensation should radiate up and/or down the forearm.

Lung-7
In the crevice on the most lateral aspect of the radius, 1.5" proximal to the transverse wrist crease, at the base of the styloid process. Between the tendons of brachioradialis and abductor pollicis longus.

Applications
Lu-7 stimulates the descending and dispersing Lung functions, circulates the Defensive Ki, expels exterior pathogenic factors, promotes sweating and opens the water passages. It also has a particular effect on the head, face and neck (it is the *command point* for this area). It also aids the Kidney function of 'grasping the Ki from the Lungs', and opens the Directing Vessel, therefore nourishing the Fluids and Yin of the whole body. Symptoms it treats include: *colds and flu* due to exterior wind-cold, *blocked nose*, acute or chronic *asthma; cough* and dry, tickly, itchy or *sore throat;* skin rashes due to heat or dryness; yin deficiency or exterior wind in the Lungs and fullness of the chest; *headache, neck pain* and *facial paralysis*; urinary retention; oedema and *swelling of the face*. Lu-7 also releases excessive emotional states such as *sadness*, depression or worry and can be used following bereavement. To aid in the cessation of smoking, combine Lu-7 with Lu-9, LI-4 and Liv-3 (acupressure should be applied to Lu-7, LI-4 and Lu-9 each time there is a craving to smoke). Combine Lu-7 with LI-4, Bl-12 and Bl-13

to treat exterior wind-cold with symptoms such as chills, runny or blocked nose, aching head and neck, or with Kd-6 (Coupled point for the Directing Vessel) and Ren-12 to treat dryness of the Lungs with symptoms including dry, unproductive cough, sore throat, dry skin and thirst.

Treatment
Acupressure is applied into the small crevice regularly until acute symptoms subside in a supine or sitting position (the latter is best if there is acute difficulty breathing). A sensation may radiate to the index finger and to the thenar eminence, and/or up the arm.

Lung-9
On the transverse wrist crease, in the depression on the radial side of the radial artery. Medial to the tendon of abductor pollicis longus.

Applications
Lu-9's primary function is to improve the circulation of Ki throughout the chest and whole body, by tonifying the chest Ki[6] and the Lung Ki. It has the effect of strengthening the cardiovascular and respiratory systems and benefiting the breathing and voice. It also nourishes the Lung Yin and fluids, clears heat and resolves phlegm. It treats most chronic and deficiency conditions of the Lungs, with symptoms including: chronic cough and asthma, weak or shallow breathing, inability to talk, weak or hoarse voice, shortness of breath, lassitude and chronic tiredness, poor circulation, spontaneous sweating, cold hands and feet, palpitations, chest pain and weak or irregular pulses. It is used to 'moisten the voice' of singers and benefit people during the process of giving up smoking.

Treatment
Lu-9 can be accessed deeply by abducting the thumb simultaneously to applying acupressure. It is most effective when treated regularly for chronic Lung problems.

Lung-10
Located with the palm facing upwards on the thenar surface of the palm, halfway along the first metacarpal bone at the junction of the skin of the palmar and dorsal surface.

Applications
Clears heat and toxicity from the Lungs, transforms phlegm heat, and benefits the throat and whole respiratory tract. Symptoms it treats include: *sore, inflamed throat* due to full heat and fire; bronchitis, fever and thirst; *cough* with thick yellow sticky or dry sputum; chest pain and nosebleed.

Treatment
Strong acupressure is most effective applied regularly until symptoms subside.

Lung-11
On the radial (lateral) side of the thumb about 0.1"[7] proximal to the corner of the nail.

Applications
Lu-11 clears heat and expels wind from the Lungs and throat and resuscitates consciousness. It is most commonly used for sore throat due to external or internal wind and heat.

Treatment
As for Lu-10 and LI-1. A strong sensation reaching the chest and face should be achieved.

THE LARGE INTESTINE CHANNEL
Brighter Yang Channel of the upper limb

Large Intestine-1
On the radial (lateral) side of the index finger approximately 0.1" proximal to the corner of the nail.

Applications
LI-1 clears both interior and exterior heat and expels wind. It is of particular benefit to the throat. It is mainly used to treat *acute pain, swelling and inflammation of the throat*. Combine LI-1 with Lu-10 and Lu-11 for *acute sore throat* due to heat in the Lungs.

Treatment
Self-acupressure or even 'biting' this point oneself is a useful first aid method for sore throat (see also Lu-11).

Large Intestine-4
In the centre of the flesh between the first and second metacarpal bones at the high point of the dorsal interosseus muscle when the thumb is adducted. It is level with the midpoint of the second metacarpal bone.

Applications
LI-4 is one of the most commonly used points with a very powerful action to clear both exterior and interior pathogenic factors, clear stagnation, relax the body and stop pain of any location. LI-4 strongly descends the Ki and is used to clear the Upper Burner, including the mouth, face, head and lungs as well as calm the mind. Because of the powerful effect it has on moving the Ki, LI-4 is known as the 'analgesia point' and is often combined with Liv-3 to treat *acute pain* and *stress* whether physical or psychological. It may also be thought of rather like an 'aspirin' for conditions such as *febrile diseases*, colds, influenza, conjunctivitis, *allergic rhinitis*, sneezing, *sinusitis* and any pain condition including *headache* (especially frontal), *toothache, sore throat, abdominal pain, dysmenorrhoea, pain in the forearm, elbow or shoulder*. It is also used for *delayed labour* or *delayed menstruation, constipation*, excessive or absent sweating, stress and tension, wind stroke, substance abuse and *addiction related problems*. LI-4 induces labour and childbirth and is therefore contraindicated during pregnancy and heavy menstrual bleeding. Combine with Lu-7 and Bl-13 for exterior wind-cold, with Liv-3 for headache and nervous tension and with Sp-6 and GB-21 to induce labour.

Treatment
Ensure that pressure is applied perpendicularly to the second metacarpal bone (the hand should be in a semi-supine, semi-prone position). For acute conditions strong acupressure is applied until symptoms subside. **Caution:** Avoid it's overuse in very deficient patients, contraindicated during pregnancy and heavy menstrual bleeding.

Large Intestine-5
On the wrist in the centre of the large depression between the tendons of extensor pollicis longus and brevis ('anatomical snuff box'). To define the 'anatomical snuff box' extend the thumb. It is in the wrist joint space between the scaphoid and radius.

Applications
LI-5 is a very important point for problems of the *wrist* and thumb. Combine with TH-4 and SI-5 for problems of the wrist

Treatment
Pressure can be applied as the thumb is extended, simultaneously with mobilising the wrist joint.

Large Intestine-10
2" below LI-11, along the line joining LI-11 and LI-5 on the extensor carpi radialis muscle.

Applications
Used for *pain*, *motor impairment*, *atrophy or paralysis* of the upper limb and shoulder. It is a major point for any chronic problem of the Large Intestine channel as it tonifies the Ki and Blood and strengthens the whole arm. It is the equivalent point of St-36 on the upper limb with which it is commonly combined to strengthen the four limbs. Combine with LI-4, LI-15 and St-38 for *frozen shoulder*.

Treatment
Pressure should be strong enough for a warmth or distending soreness to extend up and down the arm. The whole arm should feel stronger and lighter after treatment.

Large Intestine-11
Located with the elbow flexed, at the lateral end of the transverse cubital crease, midway between Lu-5 and the lateral epicondyle of the humerus between the brachioradialis and the extensor carpi radialis muscles.

Applications
LI-11 is a powerful point to clear both exterior and interior heat and wind, descend excessive yang, resolve dampness, benefit the Liver and remove Ki stagnation. It is used for exterior syndromes including symptoms such as *fever* with chills and sweating, stuffed nose, cough, *body aches* and allergies due to exterior wind-heat. Common symptoms of interior heat and wind include high *fever, headache,* red eyes, *hypertension, skin diseases* with heat and redness and *swelling of the throat.* Lymphadenopathy, goitre, cough with *profuse yellow sticky phlegm*, vomiting and jaundice are all caused by dampness, phlegm and heat in the Upper and Middle Burners, whereas abdominal pain and distension, *diarrhoea* and cystitis are due to damp heat in the lower burner. LI-11 is a major point for pain, *swelling* or *impaired movement of the elbow* and arm for which it is often combined with LI-4 and Lu-5.

Treatment
Pressure may be applied with the elbow flexed or extended. A strong aching sensation should be achieved for best results.

Large Intestine-12
In the depression just above the superior margin of the lateral epicondyle of the humerus, about 1" superolateral to LI-11. It is at the origin of the anconeus muscle slightly in front of the lateral border of the triceps brachii muscle. Locate with the elbow flexed.

Applications
Used for *elbow problems*.

Treatment
Acupressure is best applied with the elbow flexed.

Large Intestine-14
On the lateral aspect of the humerus along the line joining LI-11 to LI-15, slightly anterior and superior to the insertion of the deltoid muscle.

Applications
LI-14 is mainly used to treat pain or *impaired movement of the arm* and shoulder.

Treatment
Shiatsu is best applied in a sidelying or sitting position.

Large Intestine-15
In the anterior of the two depressions that are formed when the arm is abducted, inferior to the acromion, between the anterior and middle belly of the deltoid muscle, approximately 1" anterior to TH-I4.

Applications
LI-15 is useful in any type of *shoulder problems* manifesting along the channel pathway and is often combined with LI-4.

Treatment
Sidelying or sitting positions are best to access this point.

Large Intestine-16
On the superior aspect of the shoulder in the large depression formed between the acromial extremity of the clavicle and the scapular spine, on the trapezius muscle.

Applications
LI-16 is primarily used to treat impaired mobility and other *problems of the shoulder* and arm. It has a dispersing effect on the Ki and Blood locally and also aids the Lung function of dispersing and descending. It is also used when there is phlegm accumulation in the upper Burner causing symptoms such as pain or lymph gland *swelling of the neck* and supraclavicular area, heaviness of the chest, dyspnoea and cough.

Treatment
A sensation should radiate into the shoulder and down toward the chest. Stiffness and pain should be reduced after treatment.

Large Intestine-18
Between the two heads of the sternocleidomastoid at the level of the tip of the Adam's apple 3" lateral to the anterior midline (lateral to St-9).

Applications
LI-18 is primarily used for *pain and swelling of the throat and neck* due to phlegm or heat accumulation from febrile diseases or thyroid problems. It is also used for paralysis of the hyoglossus muscle and treats loss of voice and difficulty swallowing.

Treatment
Similar to St-9.

Large Intestine-20
In the nasolabial sulcus, at the level of the midpoint of the lateral border of the nostril.

Applications
LI-20 is a major point to unblock the nose and frontal sinuses and improve sense of smell and breathing. To treat *blocked nose*, *loss of sense of smell*, *sinusitis* or facial paralysis combine LI-20 with LI-4 and Lu-7.

Treatment
Acupressure is applied regularly until the nose has unblocked and the breathing is easier.

THE STOMACH CHANNEL
Brighter Yang Channel of the lower limb

Stomach-1
Between the eye ball and the midpoint of the infraorbital ridge, level with the centre of the pupil when the eye is focussed straight ahead.

Applications
St-1 treats many *eye problems* including redness, pain, swelling and tiredness of the eyes, twitching of the lower lid and visual impairment. It is effective for improving appearance of the eyes and surrounding area.

Treatment
Regular acupressure applied to St-1 in combination with St-2, Bl-1 and GB-1 is a very effective treatment to clear and brighten the eyes and eliminate under eye puffiness or dark circles. Acupressure is best applied with the person lying in a supine position.

Stomach-2
Directly below St-1 (approximately 0.3") in the depression of the infraorbital foramen.

Applications
St-2 has similar functions to St-1 but primarily affects the front of the cheek and nose treating conditions such as sinusitis and *facial pain*.

Treatment
Regular acupressure is necessary until symptoms subside.

Stomach-3
Below the zygomatic arch, directly below St-1 and St-2, approximately level with the lower border of the nostril.

Applications
St-3 treats problems of the centre of the face and cheeks, sinuses and nose, including *blocked nose*, *sinusitis*, rhinitis and facial pain or paralysis. It also benefits the eyes, gums and teeth.

Treatment
As for St-2.

Stomach-4
Directly below St-3, about 0.4" lateral to the corner of the mouth.

Applications
St-4 treats problems of the mouth, lips and cheek including excess salivation, eating disorders and *deviation of the mouth*. It is used to *suppress the appetite* during weight loss programmes, in which case acupressure must be applied regularly.

Treatment
As for St-2. Acupressure should be applied each time there is a food craving.

Stomach-6
In the depression at the prominence of the masseter muscle, about one finger's breadth anterosuperior to the tip of the angle of mandible. Clench the jaw to define the masseter muscle.

Applications
St-6 treats problems of the jaw, temporomandibular joint (TMJ) and cheek including: tension in the jaw, *TMJ syndrome*, clenching or *grinding of the teeth*, tension headache, toothache, *swelling of the cheeks*, parotitis, facial paralysis and pain, stiffness and pain of the neck, excessive salivation.

Treatment
Shiatsu is best in a sidelying or supine position with the head turned slightly to the side and pressure applied to one side at a time. Alternately apply acupressure simultaneously to both sides in a supine or sitting position. **Caution**, excess pressure on St-6 in a side position may cause dislocation of the TMJ.

Stomach-8
At the corner of the forehead, at the pulse of the temporal artery and the superior margin of the temporalis muscle, directly above St-7 and GB-3. It is 0.5" within the anterior hairline and 4.5" lateral to the anterior midline (Du-24). To aid location clench the jaw.

Applications
St-8 treats problems of the head and is used in cases of *headache* and *migraine* (especially if one sided); muzzy, heavy feeling in the head; *dizziness and vertigo*; mental problems and *poor concentration*. It is also used to clear the eyes and treats blurred vision, twitching of the eyelids, excessive lacrimation and *facial paralysis*.

Treatment
Pressure is best applied in a supine, side or sitting position.

Stomach-9
About 1.5" lateral to the tip of the laryngeal prominence on the anterior border of the sternocleidomastoid muscle. Between the common carotid artery and thyroid cartilage. Note that the carotid sinus is just above St-9 and the vagus nerve passes just lateral to the artery. Acupressure and massage applied to this point and surrounding tissues therefore has a powerful calming effect on the nervous system particularly aiding in the regulation of blood pressure and both heart rate and output.

Applications
This is a major point to descend excessive yang and to treat problems of the throat, thyroid gland, tongue, face, head and brain. Symptoms include: redness, swelling and pain of the throat, face and eyes, hot flushes, fever, insomnia, headache and dizziness, thyroid problems, plum stone throat, difficulty swallowing and speech impairment. St-9 is an extremely useful point for *tachycardia, palpitations, anxiety, panic attacks,* chest pain or constriction, severe pain anywhere in the body, acute asthma attack[8] and *raised blood pressure*. Pressure on St-9 increases the action of the parasympathetic division of the nervous system, relaxing the whole body, causing vasodilation and thus a decrease of blood pressure while it simultaneously lowers the heart rate and and output. It therefore is of great benefit to the blood vessels, heart and brain. It's effects are powerful and affect the entire body.

Treatment
Shiatsu is best applied in a supine position without a pillow under the head or in a sitting position. Regular acupressure applied to St-9 may be used to aid the thyroid gland, improve the metabolism, benefit the complexion and stop hot flushes. **Caution:** Great care should be taken when applying pressure to St-9. Pressure should be applied one side at a time and not both sides simultaneously.

Stomach-12
At the midpoint of the supraclavicular fossa, 4" lateral to the midline. The subclavian artery passes below St-12.

Applications

St-12 is similar to St-9 in treating excessive yang causing heat and a hyperactivity of Ki in the upper body. It also descends Ki in the chest and stomach strongly and is very effective in the treatment of *hiccup*, *dyspnoea*, cough, acute asthma attack[9], fullness of the chest, *nausea, retching,* swelling of the throat, *lymphadenopathy* and pain in the shoulder and neck.

Treatment

Shiatsu is best applied in a sitting position perpendicularly down into the chest or in a side or supine position. The pulse of the subclavian artery can be palpated when strong pressure is applied to St-12. One should have a sensation radiating down through the lungs into the chest reaching the stomach or intestine. **Caution:** Avoid overstimulation in deficient and pregnant patients, or those suffering from heart disease.

Stomach-17

In the centre of the nipple. Level with the fourth intercostal space, 4" lateral to the anterior midline. **Note:** This is a reference point and is not generally used to treat. It may however be stimulated to improve hormone levels in conditions such as amenorrhoea, infertility, uterine prolapse, loss of libido, frigidity and dysmenorrhoea.

Stomach-18

Just below the root of the breast, in the fifth intercostal space directly below the nipple, 4" lateral to the anterior midline.

Applications

St-18 is a very useful point for problems of the breasts and is used to treat pain and *swelling of the breasts*, insufficient lactation, *mastitis*, fullness or pain in the chest, asthma and cough.

Treatment

Similar to Liv-14 (located below St-18, in the sixth intercostal space). Pressure is best applied in a supine or sitting position. A sensation should radiate upwards under the breast and outwards across the chest.

Stomach-19, -20, -21, -22, -23, -24

2" lateral to Ren-14 (6" above the umbilicus), Ren-13 (5" above the umbilicus), Ren-12 (4" above the umbilicus), Ren-11 (3" above the umbilicus), Ren-10 (2" above the umbilicus) and Ren-9 (1" above the umbilicus) respectively.

Applications

All the above points benefit the stomach, abdomen and chest and are used to treat *vomiting*, *epigastric pain*, poor appetite, *abdominal distension*, intercostal neuralgia and *chest pain*. St-21 may also be considered as a Stomach Bo point for situations of a more excess type than Ren-12. It is also especially useful for descending rebellious Stomach Ki leading to nausea and vomiting.

Treatment
Similar to St-25.

Stomach-25

2" lateral to Ren-8 (centre of the umbilicus), directly below St-24.

Applications

St-25 is very commonly used in problems of the intestines to clear dampness and heat from the whole lower burner and particularly from the Large Intestine. Symptoms include *irritable bowel, diarrhoea, foul smelling stools* and *abdominal distension* and pain; but also gyneacological symptoms such as leucorrhoea, irregular menstruation and *dysmenorrhoea*. It also relieves food retention and promotes the descending of Stomach Ki and is used in cases of constipation, acute *obstruction of the intestines* and vomiting.

Treatment
Shiatsu is best applied in a supine position with the hips flexed and the legs well supported with cushions, so that the abdomen can be as relaxed as possible. Self-acupressure can also be applied in a standing or sitting position while bending the trunk forward. Moxa is very effective to clear dampness from the intestines and stop diarrhoea. **Caution:** Avoid pressure on St-25 (and other abdominal points) if the abdomen is very painful and hard in cases of severe constipation, inflammation of the abdomen or pregnancy.

Stomach-28
3" below the umbilicus, 2" lateral to Ren-4.

Applications
St-28 benefits the whole of the lower abdomen and is particularly useful in the treatment of genito-urinary problems, or problems of the reproductive organs and uterus. Symptoms include *dysuria*, haematuria, *cystitis*, urethritis, *pelvic inflammatory disease, abdominal distension,* heaviness and pain.

Treatment
Similar to St-25.

Stomach-30
2" lateral to Ren-2 (5" below the umbilicus) on the upper border and slightly lateral to the pubic tubercle, medial to the external iliac vessels.

Applications
St-30 is an important point to regulate menstruation, promote fertility, descend rebellious stomach Ki and invigorate and regulate Ki and Blood in the lower burner. It is commonly used in the treatment of *infertility* and *impotence*, spermatorrhoea, *amenorrhoea*, irregular menstruation, dysmenorrhoea, frequent miscarriage, morning sickness during pregnancy, prolapse of the uterus or rectum, haemorrhoids, lower abdominal pain, *inguinal hernia* and pain of the external genitals.

Treatment
Shiatsu is best applied in a supin position with the abdomen in a relaxed position.

Stomach-31
In the prominent depression below the hip appearing when the thigh is flexed, between the sartorius and tensor fasciae latae muscles, directly below the ASIS. Approximately level with the perineum. This is a 'large' point and may be accessed from a slightly wider area extending both upwards toward the ASIS and downward lateral to the sartorius muscle.

Applications
St-31 is a very powerful point used to benefit the hips and improve flow of Ki and Blood to the entire lower extremity. St-31 treats many hip problems including *restricted movement*, atrophy, paralysis, contraction, numbness and *pain or stiffness of the lower limb* and knees. It also treats lumbar and abdominal pain.

Treatment
Strong pressure is best applied in a supine or sidelying position with the thigh flexed. An intense sensation radiates around front of the hip and abdomen or inwards to the hip and down the leg. ST-31

may also be effectively stretched by extending the femur at the hip joint in the prone, side or seiza positions. Self stimulation with the thumbs in standing and crouching positions is an effective exercise to benefit the hips and legs.

Stomach-34
2" proximal to the laterosuperior border of the patella, between the rectus femoris and vastus lateralis muscles.

Applications
St-34 has a powerful effect on pacifying the Stomach and descending rebellious Ki, clearing obstruction from the channel and benefiting the knees. It is commonly used to treat *pain or swelling of the knees*, impaired movement of the legs, *stomach ache*, acid reflux, nausea and diarrhoea.

Treatment
Shiatsu is best applied in supine with the leg rotated slightly medially.

Stomach-35
In the large depression lateral to the patellar tendon appearing when the knee is flexed. It is in the knee joint space between the femur and tibia. This point is also called the 'lateral eye of the knee' (Xiyan).

Applications and treatment
This is a very important point used in the treatment of *knee pain*, swelling or difficulty in movement. Shiatsu is best applied in supine or side with the knee bent.

Stomach-36
On the tibialis anterior muscle, 1 finger's breadth lateral to the tibial crest, level with the lower border of the tibial tuberosity. 3" below the knee crease (approximately one palm's width) and about 1" anterior and inferior to GB-34. Dorsiflexion of the foot defines the tibialis anterior muscle.

Applications
One of the most commonly used points and a major tonifying point (it tonifies all the vital substances). It is used in most chronic conditions of deficiency of Ki, Blood, Yin or Yang and weakness of the Stomach, Spleen and other organs. Symptoms it treats include: *tiredness*, weakness, debility, feeling 'low' emotionally, spontaneous sweating, shortness of breath, *weak immunity*, recurrent colds and flus, asthma, *poor appetite*, *indigestion*, *nausea*, vomiting, *epigastric pain*, *abdominal distension*, loose stools, constipation, diarrhoea, scant menstruation, *amenorrhoea*, infertility, dry skin and hair, premature ageing, dizziness, *prolapse of organs*, *hypo or hypertension*, thirst, dry mouth, low grade fever, insomnia, palpitations, diseases of the breast, chest pain and epilepsy. St-36 benefits the tendons and can be used to stimulate athletes' muscles before and after exercising or in cases of tiredness and *weakness, atrophy or paralysis of the legs*, *knee pain* and back pain. Combine St-36 with Ren-6 to tonify the Ki, with Kd-6 and Ren-12 to nourish the Yin and fluids, with Sp-6 to nourish the Blood, with Lu-9 to tonify the Lung Ki, with St-18 and SI-1 to promote lactation and with HP-6 to stop nausea.

Treatment
Shiatsu is best applied in a supine position with the knees extended or slightly bent with a support cushion under the leg. Regular acupressure helpsto strengthen the legs and tonify the vital substances. A sensation should radiate deeply into and around the point and up and down the channel, reaching the ankle and toes or hip, abdomen and chest. Moxa is also very effective to tonify the Yang and expel cold from the Stomach.

Stomach-37
3" below St-36, 6" below the knee crease, one finger's breadth lateral to the tibial crest.

Applications
St-37 is used to clear dampness and/or heat from of the Large Intestine and is used in the treatment of *diarrhoea*, borborygmus, abdominal pain and any *acute conditions of the intestine.*

Treatment
Similar to St-36. A sensation radiating upwards has the best results. Moxa is also very effective to clear dampness from the intestine.

Stomach-38
8" below the knee crease (8" above the external malleolus), one finger's breadth lateral to the tibial crest.

Applications and treatment
Similar to St-37 and St-39. St-38 is a distal point for pain and stiffness of the shoulder.

Stomach-39
9" below the knee crease (7" above the external malleolus), one finger's breadth lateral to the tibial crest.

Applications and treatment
Similar to St-37, but affecting the Small Intestine more.

Stomach-40
In a depression on the anterolateral aspect of the leg, halfway down the leg (8" below the knee crease and 8" above the lateral malleolus). Between the extensor digitorum longus and peroneus brevis muscles, 2 finger's breadth lateral to the tibial crest (1 finger's breadth lateral to St-38).

Applications
St-40 is the main point used to resolve phlegm from any part of the body, but particularly from the digestive and respiratory systems. It also resolves dampness, clears heat, opens and relaxes the chest, calms and clears the mind. Symptoms it treats include: *productive cough*, *dyspnoea*, tightness, *heaviness or pain of the chest* or epigastrium, *vomiting*, *mental restlessness* and anxiety, depression, psychological problems, *insomnia*, *dizziness*, vertigo, muzziness and headache, *numbness* of the legs and body, lumps and cysts. Combine with Lu-1 and Lu-5 for productive cough and with Ren-12 for nausea.

Treatment
Similar to St-36; a stronger sensation is often achieved.

Stomach-41
On the front of the ankle joint, at the junction of the dorsum of the foot and the leg, in the depression between the tendons of extensor digitorum longus and extensor hallucis longus. Level with the tip of the lateral malleolus.

Applications and treatment
St-41 is a very effective point used mainly for problems of the ankle and foot including *arthritis*, *pain and swelling of the ankle* and dorsum of the foot. It is also used for clearing heat from the stomach channel with symptoms of burning epigastric pain, thirst, dizziness, headache and vertigo.

Treatment
Extend the toes to define the tendons, and dorsiflex the foot to reach pressure deeper into the point if necessary. Mobilisation techniques to open and stretch the point are also very useful, as is moxa in the case of arthritis due to cold.

Stomach-42

On the highest point of the dorsum of the foot, at the pulse of the dorsalis pedis artery, about midway between St-41 and St-43 (in the depression distal to the junction of the second and 3rd metatarsal bones). In the depression between the base of the second and third metatarsal bones and the lateral and intermediate cuneiform bones.

Applications

St-42 tonifies the Stomach and Spleen Ki and is used to treat weakness of these organs with symptoms such as *poor appetite and digestion* and tiredness. It is also used to calm the mind in cases of depression and mental restlessness as well as being of benefit to the foot.

Treatment

Acupressure is applied until a spreading sensation is achieved extending over the dorsum of the foot to the second and third toes. Mobilisation techniques applied to the bones of the foot are effective to open St-42 and it's surrounding area.

Stomach-44

Between the second and third toes, proximal to the margin of the web (at the end of the crease), distal to the second metatarsophalangeal joint.

Applications

St-44 clears heat and fire from the Stomach and has a powerful effect on the face and head, eliminates food stagnation, benefits digestion and stops pain. It is used to treat symptoms of heat in the stomach including: *burning epigastric pain*, acid reflux, *halitosis*, bleeding gums, *toothache*, inflammation of the eyes, fever, *thirst*, facial pain or paralysis and frontal *headache*.

Treatment

Stretching the toe opens St-44 and is effective to disperse excess heat. Combine St-44 with LI-4 for problems of the face and head.

Stomach-45

On the lateral side of the second toe, 0.1" proximal to the corner of the nail.

Applications

St-45 clears heat, calms the mind and clears the eyes and is used in cases of *mental restlessness, agitation* and insomnia.

THE SPLEEN CHANNEL
Greater Yin Channel of the upper limb

Spleen-1
On the medial side of the big toe, about 0.1" proximal to the base of the nail.

Applications
Sp-1 has the function of regulating the blood, dispelling stasis and stopping bleeding anywhere in the body by aiding the Spleen's functions of *'Holding the Blood'* and *'Raising of the Ki'*. It is particularly useful in treating problems of the lower burner organs including: *excessive uterine bleeding*, dysmenorrhoea, *threatened miscarriage*, *postpartum haemorrhage*, bleeding in stool or urine, chronic leucorrhoea, abdominal distension, prolapse of the uterus or rectum, *haemorrhoids*, varicose veins, and haemorrhage anywhere in the body. This is one of the most important points to stop bleeding anywhere in the body and is most effectively used for this purpose when moxa is applied. Sp-1 also clears and calms the Heart and mind and is used for symptoms including depression, dizziness, vertigo, loss of consciousness and insomnia.

Treatment
Sp-1 is used both for first aid and prevention. For first aid moxa (or acupressure), it should be used every few hours until symptoms subside.

Spleen-3
On the medial aspect of the foot, proximal and inferior to the head of the first metatarsal bone, at the junction of the skin of the plantar and dorsal surface of the foot.

Applications
Sp-3 is a powerful point to tonify the Spleen, particularly the functions of 'Transformation and Transportation of food essences and body fluids' and to strengthen the muscles, limbs and spine. It is one of the main points to resolve dampness anywhere, but especially from the digestive system. Symptoms include: *tiredness*, weakness and *heaviness* of the limbs and body, oedema, *obesity*, poor appetite, *abdominal distension* and pain, *loose stools*, diarrhoea, leucorrhoea, excessive urination, cough with profuse sputum. Sp-3 also improves mental functions and concentration and is used for *poor concentration*, mental confusion, *sleepiness*, feeling of heaviness and muzziness. For Stomach and Spleen deficiency in general combine Sp-3 with Sp-6, St-36, Bl-20 and Bl-21. For poor concentration and tiredness due to Stomach and Spleen deficiency, combine Sp-3 with St-36 and Du-20. For dampness and phlegm accumulation in the Upper and Middle Burners combine with St-40, Lu-5 and Ren-12, for dampness in the lower burner combine with Sp-6 and Sp-9.

Treatment
Shiatsu is best applied in a supine or side position with the medial aspect of the foot facing upwards. Combine pressure with mobilisation techniques to loosen the metatarsophalangeal joint of the big toe.

Spleen-4
On the medial aspect of the foot, in the depression distal and inferior to the base of the first metatarsal bone, at the junction of the skin of the plantar and dorsal surface of the foot.

Applications
This is a very effective point to regulate the flow of Ki and Blood, stop pain and dispel stasis from the stomach, heart and uterus and to regulate menstruation because it opens the Penetrating Vessel (PV). Symptoms include: *chronic or acute pain, fullness*, heaviness and distension of the chest and abdomen, *nausea* and vomiting, *morning sickness* during pregnancy, diarrhoea, *borborygmus, irregular menstruation, dysmenorrhoea*, amenorrhoea, excessive menstrual bleeding and *infertility*. Sp-4 is often combined with HP-6 (the Coupled point for the PV.).

Treatment
As for Sp-3.

Spleen-5

In the depression midway between the tuberosity of the navicular bone and the tip of the medial malleolus.

Applications

Sp-5 strengthens the Stomach and Spleen, resolves dampness and moves stagnant Ki. It is mainly used for problems of the ankle, foot, leg and knee (combine with St-41, GB-40, Liv-4), but also treats interior conditions of Ki and Blood stagnation or dampness manifesting as *abdominal distension, dysmenorrhoea,* endometriosis or constipation.

Treatment

Shiatsu is best applied in a supine or side position with the medial surface of the foot facing upwards. Combine acupressure with mobilisation techniques to loosen the joints of the foot and ankle.

Spleen-6

In the depression 3" above the prominence of the medial malleolus, between the posterior tibial border and soleus muscle. There are variations on the location of this point that are mainly based on clinical observation of where the point is felt to be most reactive (anteriorly it affects the Spleen more, posteriorly the Kidney and in the middle the Liver). It is important to feel the depression which is often larger and softer in women.

Applications

Sp-6 is one of the major points to tonify and nourish the Blood and Yin, calm and cool the whole body and strengthen the Spleen, Liver and Kidneys, whose channels converge at this point. It also resolves dampness, smooths the flow of Ki and Blood, removes stagnation, particularly from the lower burner and regulates the uterus and menstruation. Symptoms it treats include: *tiredness,* poor appetite and digestion, *abdominal distension and pain,* loose or bitty stools, constipation, irritable bowel syndrome, *impotence,* vaginal discharge, *genital itching or pain, dysuria, dysmenorrhoea, amenorrhoea, irregular or delayed menstruation, delayed and difficult labour, infertility,* dizziness, tinnitus, vertigo, *feeling of heat,* dry mouth and throat, *night sweats,* skin diseases due to heat, *restlessness, palpitations, insomnia,* weakness, atrophy or paralysis of the lower limb, *oedema.* Combine Sp-6 with St-36, Bl-20 and Bl-21 for Spleen and Stomach deficiency; with Sp-9 and Ren-3 for damp accumulation in the lower burner causing dysuria or vaginal discharge; with He-7 for insomnia and restlessness due to Blood deficiency; with Liv-3, Sp-4 and Ren-4 for dysmenorrhoea due to Ki and Blood stasis and with Kd-6 and Ren-4 to nourish the Yin.

Treatment

Shiatsu is best applied in a supine or side position with the knees slightly bent and well supported with cushions. Palm pressure is in many cases the most effective method as the thumbs may be more painful. Sp-6 is often tender in women, especially pre-menstrually. **Contraindicated** during pregnancy or heavy menstrual bleeding.

Spleen-8

5" below the knee crease (10" above the medial malleolus), on the medial belly of the soleus muscle, posterior to the border of the tibia. It is on the line connecting Sp-9 and the medial malleolus.

Applications

Sp-8 is a powerful point to regulate the flow of Ki and Blood, remove stasis and stop pain from the whole Spleen channel, abdomen and uterus. Symptoms include: acute or chronic *dysmenorrhoea, acute pain anywhere along the channel*, particularly in the knees and abdomen, retention of urine, oedema, *abnormal uterine bleeding* and seminal emissions.

Treatment
Similar to Sp-6. **Caution** Sp-8 can be very painful, care should be taken not to overstimulate it in sensitive patients.

Spleen-9
In the depression directly below the medial tibial condyle, between the medial tibial border and the gastrocnemius muscle.

Applications
Sp-9 is one of the most powerful points to drain dampness, clear heat and regulate the lower burner particularly in relation to the Intestines and genitourinary systems. Common symptoms it is used for include: *abdominal distension*, any *urinary difficulty* including urinary retention, incontinence, nephritis, urethritis and *cystitis*, *vaginal discharge*, irregular menstruation, *dysentery*, diarrhoea, mucus in the stools, *oedema* of the lower limbs and abdomen, painful and *swollen knees*, lower back ache.

Treatment
Strong pressure should be applied until a distending warmth or sore sensation extends around the point and up and down the channel. Moxa is effective to clear cold dampness.

Spleen-10
2" above the mediosuperior border of the patella, on the protuberance of the vastus medialis muscle located with the knee flexed. The 2" are measured from the patella's lower to upper borders.

Applications
Sp-10 is used to clear heat from the blood, remove blood stasis, stop bleeding, regulate menstruation and tonify the blood with it's broadest application in gyneacological and skin diseases. Symptoms include *irregular menstruation*, *dysmenorrhoea*, *excessive or abnormal uterine bleeding*, genital sores, *skin diseases* due to blood heat and stagnation including *eczema*, psoriasis, urticaria and any rash, haematuria, *pain on the inside of the thigh and knee*.

Treatment
Similar to Sp-9.

Spleen-12
In the inguinal groove, level with the upper border of the pubic symphysis, 3.5" lateral to the anterior midline on the lateral side of the femoral artery. See also Liv-12.

Spleen-13
About 0.7" superolateral to Sp-12, approximately 4" lateral to the anterior midline.

Spleen-15
On the lateral edge of the rectus abdominis muscle, approximately 4" lateral to the centre of the umbilicus.

Applications
Sp-15 is a very useful point for the treatment of many intestinal and digestive problems. It's functions are similar to those of St-25 (the Bo point for the Large Intestine), but it is used more often in the treatment of chronic, deficiency conditions. Symptoms it is used for include: *constipation* or chronic *loose stools* due to *weakness of the abdomen*, *abdominal distension*, heavy feeling, *weakness of the limbs and body*.

Treatment

As for St-25. Moxa is also effective to clear dampness from the intestines and tonify the Spleen Yang. **Caution:** Avoid pressure on Sp-15 if the abdomen is very painful and hard in cases of severe constipation, inflammation of the abdomen or pregnancy.

Spleen-16

Directly below the ribcage, at the lateral edge of the rectus abdominis muscle, approximately 4" lateral to the midline, 3" above Sp-15 (level with Ren-11 and St-22).

Spleen-17

6" lateral to Ren-16 in the fifth intercostal space.

Spleen-20

Below Lu-1, 6" lateral to the anterior midline in the second intercostal space.

Spleen-21

On the mid-axillary line, midway between He-1 and Liv-13 (midway between the centre of the axilla and free end of the 11th rib), usually found in the seventh intercostal space

Applications

Sp-21 is used to invigorate Blood, remove blood stasis and stop pain anywhere in the body or to nourish the Ki and Blood. It particularly benefits the chest, Heart, Lungs and Spleen.

Treatment

Shiatsu is best applied in a sidelying position with the palms. **Caution:** Do not apply excessively strong pressure on over deficient, elderly or heart disease patients.

THE HEART CHANNEL
Lesser Yin Channel of the upper limb

Heart-1
In the centre of the axilla, either medial to, or on the axillary artery. Locate and treat with the arm abducted above the head.

Applications
He-1 is a powerful point affecting three main areas: (a) diseases of the axillary area causing symptoms such as pain, *swelling*, lumps, skin diseases, *excessive sweating* and mastitis due to heat and fire in the Liver or Heart; (b) diseases of the Heart and blood vessels due to empty or full heat; (c) the motility of the shoulder and arm and is used in the treatment of *frozen shoulder* and inability to raise the arm.

Treatment
Shiatsu is best applied in a supine position with the arm in abduction. Palm pressure is most effective to nourish the Yin and calm the Heart, whereas stretching open the axilla in a supine or sitting position is most effective for dispersing excessive heat from the Heart or dispelling Ki and Blood stasis from the shoulder joint. **Caution**: take care not to overstimulate He-1 as it may be painful. In cases of inflamed glands or painful lumps, do not apply pressure directly to the affected area.

Heart-3
In the depression in front of the medial epicondyle of the humerus at the medial end of the transverse cubital crease. Locate with the elbow flexed.

Applications
He-3 has a calming effect on the Heart and mind as it clears both full and empty heat and resolves phlegm from the Heart. Symptoms it is commonly used for include: *depression*, psychosis, poor memory, epilepsy, *chest pain*, numbness of the forearm, *problems of the elbow* and ulnar nerve.

Treatment
Shiatsu is best applied in a supine position with the arm in abduction and the elbow flexed.

Heart-4, -5, -6, -7
On the radial side of the tendon of flexor carpi ulnaris, He-4 is 1.5" proximal to the transverse wrist crease, He-5 is 1" proximal, He-6 is 0.5" proximal and He-7 is on the transverse wrist just proximal to the pisiform bone.

Applications
He-5 is used mainly to tonify and regulate the Heart Ki, balance the heart rate and rhythm and benefit the tongue. It also has an effect on the Small Intestine being of benefit in urinary problems. Common symptoms it is used for include: *palpitations, arrhythmia*, chest pain, spontaneous sweating, *stuttering*, aphasia or other speech difficulties, sadness, fright, *shock*, hysteria, depression and other 'deficiencies' of the mind, *dysuria* and haematuria due to heat in the Small Intestine and Bladder. **He-6** is a powerful point to clear heat from the Heart, nourish the Yin and calm the mind. It is mostly used to stop *night sweating*. It is also used to regulate Heart Blood and treats symptoms such as stabbing, acute *chest pain*, fullness of the chest, coughing blood and arrhythmia. Combine He-6 with LI-4 and Kd-6 to stop night sweating and nourish the Yin. **He-7** is one of the main points to calm the mind, reduce anxiety and regulate and nourish the heart. It is primarily used in deficiency patterns of the Heart, particularly when the Blood and Yin are depleted. Common symptoms it is used for include *palpitations*, dull complexion, chest pain, *insomnia*, *anxiety*, worry, stress and *poor memory*. Combine He-7 with Sp-6, Bl-15 and Bl-17 to nourish Heart Blood.

Treatment

Shiatsu and acupressure may be applied effectively in many positions. Moxa, magnets and specially designed 'bracelets' that stimulate He-7, may be used effectively to treat palpitations, insomnia, night sweats, etc.

Heart-8

On the palm of the hand, in the depression proximal to the metacarpophalangeal joint of the fourth and fifth digits. It is usually found on the distal transverse palmar crease, known as 'the heart line' in palmistry.

Applications

Used primarily in excess conditions to clear heat and fire from the heart with symptoms such as palpitations, *tachycardia*, sore throat, thirst, tongue ulcers, dysuria.

Treatment

Apply acupressure every few hours until symptoms subside.

Heart-9

0.1" from the radial (lateral) corner of the base of the nail of the little finger.

Applications

He-9 is used to clear and calm the mind, *restore consciousness* and regulate the Heart.

THE SMALL INTESTINE CHANNEL
Greater Yang Channel of the upper limb

Small Intestine-1
On the ulnar side of the little finger, about 0.1" proximal to the corner of the nail.

Applications
SI-1 is used to release exterior wind-heat, calm the mind and restore consciousness, benefit the breasts and promote lactation.

Small Intestine-3
On the ulnar aspect of the hand, in the depression proximal to the head ofthe fifth metacarpal bone, at the junction of the palmar and dorsal skin. At the end of the distal transverse palmar crease (known as the 'heart line'). To aid location make a loose fist.

Applications
SI-3 is used to clear wind and heat both from the exteriorand the interior, to tonify and regulate the Yang Ki and benefit the spine (especially the neck) by opening the Governing Vessel. It also calms the mind. Symptoms it treats include: *stiffness and pain of the neck*, upper back and shoulders, aching and stiffness of the spine, pain of the elbow and wrist, *headache* (particularly occipital), chills and fever, tinnitus, inflammation of the eyes, *dizziness*, hypertension, insomnia and epilepsy. Combine with Du-14 for pain and stiffness of the neck or with Bl-62 (Coupled point for the Governing Vessel) to treat unilateral pain, stiffness or paralysis of the limbs or trunk.

Treatment
Strong acupressure is applied regularly until acute symptoms subside. Techniques that stretch and open the ulnar side of the hand are also effective to disperse pathogenic factors such as wind and heat. A sore distending sensation should be achieved radiating around the point and up the channel.

Small Intestine-6
On the posterior aspect of the head of ulna, in the bony cleft (between the tendons of extensor carpi ulnaris and extensor digiti minimi) appearing when the palm faces the chest (supination of the forearm). To aid location place your index finger on the head of ulna and slowly turn the palm toward the chest so as to feel the cleft between the tendons. Extending the little finger and wrist defines the tendons.

Applications
SI-6 is a particularly effective point to *stop pain* anywhere along the Small Intestine channel, particularly the wrist and elbow.

Small Intestine-8
Located with the elbow flexed in the shallow depression of the flat area between the olecranon process of the ulna and the medial epicondyle of the humerus.

Applications
SI-8 is an effective point for *problems of the ulnar nerve, elbow, forearm and shoulder*.

Treatment
Strong acupressure or moxa is applied regularly until symptoms subside. Stretching SI-8 in a sitting or supine position is also effective.

Small Intestine-9
On the posterior aspect of the shoulder, 1" above the end of the axillary fold on the teres major muscle.

Located with the arm in a relaxed position hanging freely down by the side of the body, below the posterior border of the deltoid muscle at the lateral margin of the scapula.

Applications and treatment
See SI-11

Small Intestine-10
Directly above SI-9, in the depression directly below the scapular spine on the deltoid muscle, directly superior to the posterior axilliary crease when the arm in a relaxed position hanging freely down by the side.

Applications and treatment
See SI-11

Small Intestine-11
In the centre of the scapula. Midway between the medial and lateral border, one-third of the distance along the line joining the midpoint of the of the lower border of the scapular spine to the inferior angle of scapula. SI-11 may be accessed from a wider area covering the entire centre of the scapula, where it is felt to be most reactive.

Applications
SI-9, SI-10, SI-11 and SI-12 are all very useful points for many problems of the *shoulder and arm*. They are primarily used to treat *impaired mobility* (particularly with difficulty in adduction), *paralysis, pain or inflammation of the shoulder and arm*. SI-11 is probably the most commonly used of these four points having a very powerful relaxing effect on the whole shoulder. SI-11, -12, -13 and -14 also have a calming and relaxing effect on the digestive system, particularly the stomach, oesophagus, intestine, liver and gall bladder when there are symptoms such as indigestion, abdominal pain, irritable bowel, diarrhoea, dysphagia, hypochondrial pain and acid reflux.

Treatment
Pressure is applied deep into the joint spaces with the arm in various positions (depending on flexibility of shoulder). Treatment is best applied in a sitting or side position so that the shoulder can bemoved freely, although shiatsu can also be given in a prone position. Mobilisation techniques, combined with stretching the arm and shoulder at various angles to release stagnation from the points is most effective. Moxa and cupping is very successful in the treatment of *frozen shoulder* and stiffness due to cold and stasis of Blood. Do not apply moxa if there is inflammation of the shoulder joint capsule (cups may be applied to clear the heat, dampness and stagnation of Ki and Blood of the inflammation). Pain and stiffness should be reduced after treatment.

Small Intestine-12
In the centre of the suprascapular fossa, directly above SI-11, about 1"superior to the mid-point of the upper border of the scapular spine. A depression is formed when the arm is abducted.

Applications and treatment
See SI-11.

Small Intestine-13
At the medial end of the suprascapular fossa, aboutmidway between SI-10 and the spinous process of the second thoracic vertebra.

Applications and treatment
See SI-14.

Small Intestine-14
3" lateral to the lower border of the spinous process of the first thoracic vertebra (Du-13)on the line of the medial border of scapula (i.e., the outer Bladder channel line).

Applications
SI-13 and SI-14 (similarly to SI-9, SI-10, SI-11) all effectively improve the flow of Ki and Blood and *stop pain of the shoulder and arm but also of the upper back and neck.*

Treatment
Shiatsu, acupressure, cupping and/or moxa should be applied until an aching sensation spreading in the surrounding area is achieved. Pain and stiffness should be diminished after the treatment, which is best applied in a sitting or side position. (See also SI-11).

Small Intestine-15
2" lateral to the lower border of C7 (Du-14), at the end of the transverse process of T1.

Applications
SI-15 is used to treat problems of the neck, shoulder, upper limb and lungs, *stiffness of the neck*, asthma, *cough* and bronchitis. (See also SI-14).

Treatment
As for SI-14.

Small Intestine-17
In the depression immediately posterior to the angle of mandible, on the anterior border of sternocleidomastoid.

Applications
SI-17 is an effective point for problems of the ear, cheek, throat and tongue.

Treatment
Acupressure should be applied until a sore, distending sensation radiates to the affected areas.

Small Intestine-18
In the depression on the lower border of the zygomatic arch, directly below the outer canthus of the eye.

Applications
SI-18 is effectivefor problems of the cheeks, eyes and teeth, including inflammatory conditions such as sinusitis, otitis, parotitis and swelling of the cheeks.

Treatment
Regular acupressure should be applied until symptoms subside.

Small Intestine-19
Anterior to the tragus of the ear in the depression formed when the mouth is opened, above GB-2 and below TH-21.

Applications
SI-19 is very effective for many problems of the ears including *acute inflammation* (see also GB-2 and TH-21). Combine it with other local points such as GB-2, TH-21, TH-17 and SI-17 and distal points such as TH-3 and GB-43.

THE BLADDER CHANNEL
Greater Yang Channel of the lower limb

Bladder-1
1" superior to the inner canthus, locate with the eyes closed.

Applications
Bl-1 is used to clear and brighten the eyes and head as well as tonify the Yin. Symptoms include *tired, dry, inflamed eyes* and *migraine*.

Treatment
Regular acupressure is necessary when treating any chronic eyeproblem. See also St-1.

Bladder-2
At the medial end of the eyebrow, in the supraorbital notch.

Applications
Bl-2 is a very useful point for the forehead and eyes and is used for symptoms such as *frontal headache*, migraine with *pain in the eyes* and facial paralysis.

Treatment
As for Bl-1.

Bladder-10
On the lateral side of the trapezius muscle, 0.5" within the posterior hairline, approximately 1.3" lateral to Du-15 (which is above the spinous process of the C1 vertebra).

Applications
Bl-10 is a very important point to treat the neck, upperback, head and whole 'Greater Yang area'. It is used to expel exterior wind with symptoms such as *occipital headache*, pain and *inflammation of the eyes*, *stiffness of the neck* and *dizziness*.

Treatment
Shiatsu is best applied in a supine position (without a cushion) or sitting up. See also GB-20. **Caution:** Avoid excessive pressure on the neck.

Bladder-11
1.5" lateral to the lower border of the spinous process of the first thoracic vertebra. All the points of the inner Bladder channel line are located on the highest part of the sacrospinalis muscle group, at a distance measured halfway between the posterior midline and medial border of the scapula on the thorax. For the lower lumbar and sacral points, the 1.5" distance is measured from the medial border of the PSIS to the posterior midline. In general the locations of these points vary to a degree, being slightly further lateral in the mid-thoracic area which is often broader, or when there is deformity of the spine and thorax in cases such as kyphosis or scoliosis of the spine. They should therefore always be located where they are felt to be most reactive on palpation. A sensation spreading into the pertaining organs/areas of the body should be felt on sustained pressure. Alternatively or additionally, they may be located in the groove running next to the spine, 0.5" lateral to the posterior midline (these points are also known as the Huatuo points).

Applications
Bl-11 is the *Gathering point for Bones* and one of the points of the *'Sea of Blood'*. It is used to treat problems of the bones, spine and Blood. It is used to assist the healing of bone after a fracture and to treat any bone diseases including *osteoporosis* and *kyphosis of the spine*, especially if due to weakness

of the Kidney Essence and Blood. It is often combined with Bl-23 (the Kidney Yu point) and GB-39 to strengthen the Essence and Blood. It also releases the exterior, regulates Lung Ki and stops cough.

Treatment
Shiatsu is best applied in a prone position with a cushion under the chest and abdomen if necessary. A sitting or sidelying position may also be used. Moxa or cupping is effectively used to treat most points of the back in cases of Ki and Blood stasis, interior or exterior cold and deficiency of Ki and Blood. **Caution:** avoid excessive pressure on the rib cage, especially in the elderly, those suffering from heart disease, osteoporosis or asthma.

Bladder-12
1.5" lateral to the lower border of the spinous process of the second thoracic vertebra. See also Bl-11.

Applications
Similar to Bl-13 but used more for acute and exterior Lung problems.

Treatment
See Bl-11.

Bladder-13
1.5" lateral to the lower border of the spinous process of T3. See also Bl-11.

Applications
Bl-13 is the *Yu point for the Lung* and is used for both interior and exterior Lung problems. Treatment See Bl-11.

Bladder-14
1.5" lateral to the lower border of the spinous process of T4. See alsoBl-11.

Applications
Bl-14 is the *Yu point for the Heart Protector* (Absolute Yin Yu point).

Treatment
See Bl-11.

Bladder-15
1.5" lateral to the lower border of the spinous process of T5. See also Bl-11.

Applications
Bl-15 is the *Yu point for the Heart*.

Treatment
See Bl-11.

Bladder-16
1.5" lateral to the lower border of the spinous process of T6. See also Bl-11.

Applications
Bl-16 is the *Yu point for the Governing Vessel*.

Treatment
See Bl-11.

Bladder-17

1.5" lateral to the lower border of the spinous process of T7. See also Bl-11.

Applications
Bl-17 is the *Yu point for the Diaphragm* and *Gathering point for Blood*.

Treatment
See Bl-11. Moxa is used to nourish the Blood whereas a dispersing stimulation dispels Blood stasis.

Bladder-18

1.5" lateral to the lower border of the spinous process of T9. See also Bl-11.

Applications
Bl-18 is the *Yu point for the Liver*.

Treatment
See Bl-11.

Bladder-19

1.5" lateral to the lower border of the spinous process of T10. See also Bl-11.

Applications
Bl-19 is the *Yu point for the Gallbladder*.

Treatment
See Bl-11.

Bladder-20

1.5" lateral to the lower border of the spinous process of T11. See also Bl-11.

Applications
Bl-20 is the *Yu point for the Spleen*.

Treatment
See Bl-11.

Bladder-21

1.5" lateral to the lower border of the spinous process of T12.

Applications
Bl-21 is the *Yu point for the Stomach*.

Treatment
See Bl-11.

Bladder-22

1.5" lateral to the lower border of the spinous process of L1.

Applications
Bl-22 is the *Yu point for the Triple Heater*.

Treatment
See Bl-11.

Bladder-23
1.5" lateral to the lower border of the spinous process of L2.

Applications
Bl-23 is the *Yu point for the Kidney*.

Treatment
See Bl-11. **Caution:** avoid excessive pressure on the lumbar area, particularly in the elderly or those suffering from asthma. During pregnancy great care should be taken and only very light pressure can be applied. Conversely, very robust people may require stronger pressure, which may be carefully applied with the elbows.

Bladder-24
1.5" lateral to the lower border of the spinous process of L3.

Applications
Bl-24 is the *Yu point for the Sea of Ki*.[10]

Treatment
See Bl-11.

Bladder-25
1.5" lateral to the lower border of the spinous process of L4.

Applications
Bl-25 is the *Yu point for the Large Intestine*.

Treatment
See Bl-11.

Bladder-26
1.5" lateral to the lower border of the spinous process of L5.

Applications
Bl-26 is the *Yu point for the Original Ki Gate*.[11]

Treatment
See Bl-11.

Bladder-27
Level with the first sacral foramen (Bl-31), 1.5" lateral to the posterior midline. The 1.5" can be measured from the medial border of the PSIS to the posterior midline.

Applications
Bl-27 is the *Yu point for the Small Intestine*.

Treatment
See Bl-11.

Bladder-28
Level with the second sacral foramen (Bl-32), 1.5" lateral to the posterior midline.

Applications
Bl-28 is the *Yu point for the Bladder*.

Treatment
See Bl-11.

Bladder-29
At the level of the third sacral foramen, 1.5 lateral to the posterior midline.

Applications
Bl-29 is the *Yu point for the backbone*.[12]

Treatment
See Bl-11.

Bladder-30
At the level of the fourth sacral foramen, 1.5 lateral to the posterior midline.

Applications
Bl-30 is the *Yu point for the anus*.[13]

Treatment
See Bl-11.

Bladder-31, -32, -33, -34
In the first, second, third and fourth sacral foramina respectively, 1.5" lateral to the posterior midline.

Bladder-36
In the middle of the transverse gluteal fold, lateral to the tendon of the biceps femoris muscle.

Bladder-39
On the transverse popliteal crease, on the medial side of the biceps femoris tendon (lateral to Bl-40).

Applications
Bl-39 is the Lower Sea point of the Triple Heater.

Bladder-40
At the midpoint of the transverse popliteal crease, midway between the tendons of the biceps femoris and the semitendinosus muscles; located in prone position with the knee flexed.

Applications
Bl-40 is the Command point for the back and is used to treat back problems of both acute and chronic nature. Combine Bl-40 with local pain points to treat *acute back ache* and with points to strengthen the the spine and Kidney Ki such as Bl-23, Bl-52, Kd-3 and Du-4 for chronic lower backache.

Treatment
Since Bl-40 is one of the most important points used for back pain there is a wide variety of techniques that can be applied to it. Apart from the obvious techniques in a prone position (careful shiatsu should be applied to the entire popliteal fossa) the shiatsu practitioner can also carefully apply pressure in a supine position with the person's knee bent. Pain and stiffness should be diminished after treatment. **Caution**: Distended blood vessels are common in the popliteal area.

Bladder-42
Below Bl-47, 3" lateral to the lower border of the spinous process of T3. All the outer Yu points should be located in the intercostal spaces (not on the ribs).

Applications
Bl-47 is considered to be the *Yu point for the Corporeal Soul* (Po) and is used mainly to treat psychological problems due to disharmony of the Corporeal Soul, Lungs and Metal Element in general. The name of this point means 'Door of the Po'.

Treatment
See Bl-11.

Bladder-43
Below Bl-42, 3" lateral to the lower border of the spinous process of T4.

Applications
Bl-43 is used to treat any chronic, serious diseases particularly if affecting the chest.

Treatment
See Bl-11.

Bladder-44
3" lateral to the lower border of the spinous process of T5.

Applications
Bl-44 is considered to be the *Yu point for the Mind (Shen)* and is used mainly to treat psychological problems relating to disharmony of the Heart and all aspects and levels of consciousness, especially on an emotional and 'psycho-spiritual' level. The name of this point means '*Spirit's Hall*'.

Treatment
See Bl-11.

Bladder-47
3" lateral to the lower border of the spinous process of T9.

Applications
Bl-47 is considered to be the *Yu point for the Ethereal Soul (Hun)* and is used mainly to treat psychological problems relating to disharmony of the the Ethereal Soul and imbalances of the Liver and Wood Element in general. The name of this point means 'Gate of the Hun'.

Treatment
See Bl-11.

Bladder-49
3" lateral to the lower border of the spinous process of T11.

Applications
Bl-49 is considered to be the *Yu point for Thought (Yi)* and is primarily employed in the treatment of psychological problems relating to disharmony of the Spleen and the Earth Element in general, particularly in relation to mental processes. The name of this point means '*Abode of Thought*'.

Treatment
See Bl-11.

Bladder-52

3" lateral to the lower border of the spinous process of L2.

Applications

Bl-52 is considered to be the *Yu point for Willpower (Zhi)* and is used to treat Kidney deficiency and psychological problems relating to disharmony of the Kidneys and the willpower. The name of this point means *'Will's Chamber'*.

Treatment

Similar to Bl-23.

Bladder-54

On the highest point of the buttock, level with the sacral hiatus, 3" lateral to the posterior midline.

Applications

Bl-54 is a very effective local point for the treatment of pain of the lower back and buttocks, including sciatic, pelvic or anal pain.

Treatment

Shiatsu is best applied in a prone or sidelying position with the palms, forearms, knees or feet.

Bladder-56

In the centre of the gastrocnemius muscle, between the two heads, midway between Bl-55 and Bl-57.

Applications and treatment

Similar to Bl-57.

Bladder-57

On the posterior aspect of the calf, directly below the body of gastrocnemius muscle, approximately 8" below Bl-40, (halfway between Bl-40 to Bl-60) along the line joining Bl-40 with the insertion of the achilles tendon.

Applications

Bl-57 is a primary point for problems of the channel pathway (particularly the calf) and is commonly used if there is pain, cramps or weakness of the calf and leg, sciatica or lumbar pain. In addition it also treats interior conditions such as haemorrhoids, pain of the perineum or anus and dysmenorrhoea.

Treatment

Pressure should be applied carefully (light palm pressure may be best initially) as the whole area can often be very sensitive, tight and painful. **Caution**: Avoid pressure on distended blood vessels or inflamed areas.

Bladder-58

On the posterior aspect of the calf, approximately 1" inferolateral to Bl-57, between the posterior border of fibula and the anterolateral border of the gastrocnemius muscle, 7" above the tip of the external malleolus.

Bladder-60

On the outside of the ankle, in the centre of the noticeable depression, between the posterior border of the external malleolus and the anterior border of the achilles tendon, level with the tip of the external malleolus when the foot is at right angles.

Applications

Bl-60 is a useful point in the treatment of back pain or any obstruction along the pathway of the Bladder channel. It also tonifies the Kidneys as it is so close to Kd-3 (located opposite Bl-60 on the inner aspect of the ankle).

Treatment

In general, thumb or finger pressure is best in order to locate the point precisely. A sensation should travel up the outer aspect of the leg.

Bladder-61

On the lateral aspect of the foot, below Bl-60, in the depression of the calcaneum, at the junction of the skin of the plantar and dorsal aspects of the foot.

Bladder-62

In the depression directly below the tip of the external malleolus, approximately 0.5" below the inferior border (opposite to Kd-6).

Applications

Bl-62 is the *Opening point of the Yang Heel Vessel* and has the function of regulating the flow of Yang Ki and descending excessive Yang. In a sense, Bl-62 has opposite functions to Kd-6 which opens the Yin Heel Vessel and has the function of increasing the Yin Ki. Combine with TH-5 to treat unilateral pain or stiffness due obstruction of the Yang Heel Vessel.

Treatment

Similar to Bl-60.

Bladder-64

On the lateral aspect of the dorsum of the foot, in the depression proximal to the tuberosity of the fifth metatarsal bone, at the junction of the skin of the plantar and dorsal aspects of the foot.

Bladder-65

On the lateral aspect of the dorsum of the foot, proximal to the head of the fifth metatarsal bone, at the junction of the skin of the plantar and dorsal aspects of the foot.

Bladder-67

On the lateral aspect of the small toe, about 0.1" proximal to the nail.

Applications

Bl-67 has a powerful effect on the uterus by activating the Yang Ki of the Bladder and Kidney. It is therefore **contraindicated during pregnancy.** However, in the case of breach presentation the application of moxa is employed to turn the foetus in the seventh and eighth month. It is also used to induce labour and expedite delivery of the baby and placenta.

Treatment

Moxa is applied once or twice daily for at about 15 minutes until the foetus takes position. **Caution**: discontinue moxibustion as soon as the foetus has turned.

THE KIDNEY CHANNEL
Lesser Yin channel of the lower limb

Kidney-1

On the sole of the foot, one third of the distance from the base of the toes to the heel, in the depression between the second and third metatarsal bones. Locate with the foot in plantarflexion.

Applications

Kd-1 has a powerful descending effect and clears heat, fire, excessive Yang and wind of both empty and full nature. It is, however, mostly used in excess conditions, particularly when the upper body is affected. Symptoms it treats include: *headache* on the vertex or whole head, *dizziness*, vertigo, *hypertension*, *insomnia*, *mental agitation*, night sweats, stroke, coma, difficulty urinating, sciatica, *pain of the lower back*, abdomen and sole of the foot.

Treatment

Shiatsu is best applied in a prone position, either with the thumbs, elbows, knees or feet. Do not overstimulate on very weak or over deficient patients. Regular pressure or massage applied to the sole of the foot with a ball or other specially designed object for this purpose is an effective self treatment for the above mentioned key symptoms.

Kidney-3

In the depression between the posterior border of the medial malleolus and the anterior border of achilles tendon. It is level with the tip of the medial malleolus when the foot is at right angles.

Applications

Kd-3 is a major tonifying point for the Kidneys as it augments the Kidney Yin, Yang and Essence. It is of particular importance in the treatment of problems of the lower burner, particularly the Kidneys, Bladder, reproductive organs and spine. It is used in the treatment of any chronic diseases as it tonifies the Original Ki (Source Ki) which stems from the Kidney Yin and Yang. Symptoms it treats include: *exhaustion*, *diminished hearing and sight*, tinnitus, *dizziness*, sore throat, *infertility*, *impotence*, premature ejaculation, *amenorrhoea*, *irregular menstruation*, *menopausal syndromes*, *frequent or dribbling urination*, oedema, asthma due to Kidney and Lung deficiency, coldness and weakness of the lower back and abdomen, knees and legs. Combine Kd-3 with St-36 and Ren-6 to tonify the Ki and Yang of the whole body, with Bl-23 and Du-4 for chronic back ache and with Ren-4 and Sp-6 for irregular menstruation and infertility.

Treatment

Similar to Kd-2. The application of moxa is very effective to warm and activate the Kidney Yang.

Kidney-6

In the depression approximately 1" below the tip of the medial malleolus between the two tendons (define them by plantarflexing and inverting the foot). If inadequate stimulation is achieved at this location, or if the tendons are very stiff and tight, an alternative location is in the deeper depression below the sustentaculum tali. The Shiatsu practitioner can access Kd-6 successfully in a larger area covering the whole of the inner aspect of the calcaneum.

Applications

Kd-6 is one of the most important points used to nourish and moisten the Yin, cool the whole body and clear empty heat when there are symptoms such as: *night sweating*, *sore throat*, *insomnia*, restlessness, exhaustion, soreness of the lower back, premature ejaculation, *hot flushes*, *menopausal syndromes*, dryness and pain of the eyes, photophobia, diminishing vision, *tinnitus* and dizziness. Kd-6 is an important point touse in the treatment of gynaecological complaints such as *infertility*, irregular menstruation, amenorrhoea, *excessive menstrual bleeding*, genital itching and dryness, especially if combined with points such as Sp-6 and Ren-4 which support the functions of the organs of the lower burner and nourish the Yin.

Treatment

Shiatsu is best applied in a supine or side position. Long sustained pressure should be used to nourish the Yin and cool the body.

Kidney-7

2" above Kd-3 on the anterior border of the achilles tendon, along the line joining Kd-3 to Kd-10.

Applications

Kd-7 is a very important point to tonify the Yang of the Kidneys and help the water metabolism of the body thus regulating sweat, urination and movement of interstitial fluids. It is used to treat *oedema, frequent urination*, dribbling urination, anuria, lower backache, *spontaneous, excessive or lack of sweating* (combined with LI-4), abdominal distension and diarrhoea.

Treatment

Similar to Kd-3. Moxa may be used effectively.

Kidney-9

5" above Kd-3, below the belly of the gastrocnemius muscle, just anterior to the medial border of the achilles tendon. It is on the soleus muscle approximately 1" posterior to Liv-5, along the line joining Kd-3 to Kd-10.

Applications

Kd-9 clears excessive heat and phlegm while tonifying the Kidney Yin and Essence, and calming the mind. It is used to treat insomnia, psychosis, seizures, vomiting, oppression of the chest, palpitations, *inflammation of the kidneys, bladder and uterus and spasm of the calf muscles.*

Treatment

Similar to Sp-6, Liv-5 and other points of the lower calf.

Kidney-10

At the medial end of the popliteal crease between the tendons of the semitendinosus and semimembranosus muscles, level with Bl-40 and Liv-8. Locate with the knee slightly flexed.

Applications

Kd-10 transforms dampness, clears heat, tonifies the Yin and benefits the lower burner. It is used to treat symptoms such as *dysuria*, haematuria, frequent urination, chronic leucorrhoea, functional uterine bleeding and pain of the lower back and knees.

Treatment

Shiatsu is best applied in a prone or side position. The space between the two tendons is often tight and painful so pressure can be applied slightly proximal to the popliteal crease. The muscles can also be stretched and pressed to relax them so that the point opens up more easily. A tingling sensation is often felt spreading up and down the channel and into the knee.

Kidney-11

On the superior border of the pubic symphysis, 0.5" lateral to Ren-2, 5" below the umbilicus.

Applications and treatment

Similar to Ren-2, St-30 and other points of the lower abdomen. Shiatsu is applied to Kd-11 in a supine position to benefit the lower burner. It is particularly used to treat symptoms such as genital pain, urinary retention and impotence.

Kidney-16
At the centre of the abdomen, 0.5" lateral to the centre of the umbilicus (Ren-8).

Applications and treatment
Similar to Ren-8.

Kidney-21
On the epigastrium, 0.5" lateral to the anterior midline (Ren-14), 6" above the umbilicus.

Applications and treatment
Similar to Ren-14 and St-19.

Kidney-22
In the fifth intercostal space, 2" lateral to Ren-16.

Applications and treatment
Similar to Kd-25.

Kidney-25
In the second intercostal space, 2" lateral to Ren-19.

Applications
Kd-25 is especially effective in the treatment of tightness, pain and *constriction of the chest*, hiccup, *palpitations*, *asthma* and cough due to imbalances of the energetic relationships between the Kidneys, Lungs and Heart.

Treatment
Acupressure is best applied regularly in a sitting position until symptoms subside. Shiatsu may also be applied in a supine or sidelying position. Ensure the pressure is applied at the correct angle in the intercostal spaces as they are often tight and painful. **Caution**: Avoid excessive pressure on the thorax, particularly on patients with heart disease, asthma or osteoporosis.

Kidney-27
In the depression below the medial end of the clavicle, 2" lateral to the midline.

Applications and treatment
Similar to Kd-25. It also has an effect on the throat and aids the whole respiratory system by relaxing the upper thorax and neck.

THE HEART PROTECTOR CHANNEL
Absolute Yin Channel of the upper limb

Heart Protector-1
1" superolateral to the centre of the nipple, in the fourth intercostal space.

Applications
HP-1 is used to treat problems of the breasts and chest, particularly when there is Ki and Blood stagnation.

Treatment
Shiatsu applied perpendicularly to the thoracic curve with the palms (or lightly with fingertips) is best when the patient is in a supine or side position. Pressure can also be applied to the thorax under the mammary gland. **Caution**: avoid excessive pressure, as the area may be tender.

Heart Protector-2
In the centre of the upper arm, between the two heads of the biceps muscle, 2" below the anterior axillary fold.

Heart Protector-3
On the transverse cubital crease, on the lateral (ulnar) side of the tendon of the biceps brachii muscle.

Applications
HP-3 is used to clear heat from the Ki and Blood, dispel stasis and descend rebellious Ki when there are symptoms such as *chest pain*, *palpitations*, tachycardia, *dyspnoea*, cough, coughing blood, *vomiting*, convulsions, insomnia, heat stroke and *febrile diseases.*

Treatment
Shiatsu is best applied in a supine position with the arm abducted and the elbow slightly flexed so as to define the biceps brachii tendon.

Heart Protector-4
On the anterior aspect of the forearm, 5" above HP-7 at the transverse wrist crease, between the tendons of palmaris longus and flexor carpi radialis, along the line joining HP-7 with HP-3.

Applications
HP-4 has the function of cooling the Blood, dispelling stasis and stopping pain because it is the *Accumulation point* for the Heart Protector. At the same time it calms and nourishes the Heart and mind. It is used in conditions such as *pain of the chest and heart, arrhythmia,* palpitations, vomiting, *skin diseases* due to heat and stasis of the Blood, nosebleed, insomnia, fear, fright or feeling 'low' due to weakness of the Shen.

Treatment
Similar to HP-6.

Heart Protector-5
3" above the transverse wrist crease, between the tendons of palmaris longus and flexor carpi radialis.

Applications
HP-5 regulates the Ki of the chest, resolves phlegm, clears heat and calms the mind. Similar to other points of this channel (particularly HP-6) it also descends rebellious Ki and harmonises the Stomach. Symptoms it is commonly used for include *chest pain*, palpitations, cough, stomach ache, *vomiting*,

malaria, tidal fever, convulsions, epilepsy, insomnia, tongue ulcers, psychosis and *hysteria*. HP-5 may also be used to regulate menstruation.

Treatment
Similar to HP-6.

Heart Protector-6
2" above the transverse wrist crease, between the tendons of palmaris longus and flexor carpi radialis.

Applications
HP-6 is a very important point used in a wide variety of conditions. Firstly, it regulates the circulation of Ki and Blood throughout the three Burners, particularly the Triple Heater and terminal Yin channels.[14] It dispels stasis and clears heat, having a particularly powerful effect on relaxing the chest and calming the mind. Symptoms it is used for include *chest pain and constriction, palpitations, cough*, fever, *insomnia, anxiety*, irritability, *hypochondrial pain, PMS, pain of the breasts*, irregular menstruation, dysmenorrhoea, occipital headache and neck pain. Secondly, it descends rebellious Ki and harmonises the Stomach, and is a major point in the treatment of *nausea, hiccup, epigastric pain, vomiting and morning sickness during pregnancy.*

Treatment
Pressure is best applied using the thumbs or fingers to locate the point precisely. The recipient's forearm should be in supination. A sore, distending sensation (often described as 'electric') is felt radiating down and/or up the channel to the fingers and/or elbow, upper arm and chest.

Heart Protector-7
In the depression in the middle of the transverse wrist crease between the tendons of palmaris longus and flexor carpi radialis.

Applications
HP-7 has the function of clearing heat when there are symptoms such as anxiety, tachycardia, fever and scant dark urination. It descends rebellious Ki, *stops nausea, calms the mind*, relaxes the Heart and opens the chest. It's primary use is in *emotional disorders.*

Treatment
Extend the wrist slightly to expose the point.

Heart Protector-8
On the palm of the hand between the second and 3rd metacarpal bones, on the radial side of the third metacarpal bone, proximal to the metacarpophalangeal joint. When the fist is clenched, the point is just below the tip of the middle finger.

Applications
HP-8 strongly clears heat and fire from the Heart, subdues wind and calms the mind. It treats *agitation, excessive sweating, fever,* delirium, *loss of consciousness*, convulsions, nosebleed, *ulceration of the mouth and tongue*, swelling of the throat, nausea, halitosis, *palpitations* and *chest pain*. HP-8 is also extensively used in Qigong and oriental bodywork methods as a point to focus and strengthen the Ki so as to then emit or project it to the patient during the treatment. HP-8 is often combined with Kd-1.

Treatment
Acupressure is applied regularly until symptoms subside. The centre of the palm may also be stretched open to disperse and clear heat in cases of excess.

Heart Protector-9
At the centre of the tip of the middle finger, **or** 0.1" proximal to the corner of the nail on the radial side of the middle finger.

Applications
HP-9, similar to the other well points has the function of clearing heat, subduing interior wind and restoring consciousness.

Treatment
Pressure is applied onto the tip of the middle phalanx.

THE TRIPLE HEATER CHANNEL
Lesser Yang channel of the upper limb

Triple Heater-1

On the ulnar (medial) side of the fourth finger, about 0.1" proximal to the corner of the nail.

Applications

TH-1 is mainly used to clear exterior heat and wind causing symptoms such as *earache* and sore throat.

Triple Heater-4

On the dorsal aspect of the wrist, between the ulna and carpal bones, in the depression lateral to the tendon of extensor digitorum communis. Locate with the forearm in supination.

Applications

TH-4 is most commonly used to clear the channel pathway of blockages and relax the 'sinews' in the treatment of *pain, loss of motility or swelling of the hand, wrist,* elbow, shoulder and anywhere along the channel. Additionally, it clears exterior and interior heat and treats inflammatory conditions such as tonsillitis, fever, headache, thirst, inflammation of the eyes and ears, *inflammation and swelling of the joints*. It also benefits the Original Ki, the Penetrating Vessel and the Kidneys, and aids in the transformation of fluids in conditions such as: *weakness* and exhaustion, wasting syndromes, amenorrhoea, fluid retention and *oedema*.

Treatment

Extending the receiver's wrist as pressure is applied enables us to obtain a deeper pressure into the joint space. Stretching open this point in combination with mobilisation of the wrist is very effective to clear the channel pathway of obstructions.

Triple Heater-5

Between the radius and ulna, 2" above TH-4, on the radial edge of the extensor digitorum muscle.

Applications

TH-5 is a powerful point to release the exterior and expel wind-heat, remove Ki stagnation, smooth the Liver, clear interior heat and descend excessive Yang. Common symptoms it is used for include: *chills and fever* due to febrile diseases or Ki stagnation, *colds and flu*, sore throat, *stiffness and pain of the arm, shoulder and neck, hemiplegia*, irritability, hypochondrial pain, *headache and migraine, inflammation of the ears, tinnitus*, deafness, inflamed eyes. TH-5 opens the Yang Linking Vessel

Treatment

Pressure is applied either on, or just radial to, the extensor digitorum muscle. A strong sensation should be felt deep in the muscles of the forearm radiating up and/or down the arm. Pressure is applied with the receiver's forearm in supination so that theradius is parallel to the ulna (similarly to the other Triple Heater points of the forearm).

Triple Heater-6

Between the radius and ulna, close to the border of the radius, 3" above TH-4, one quarter of the distance between TH-4 and the lateral epicondyle of the humerus.

Applications

TH-6 has the functions of smoothing the flow of Ki and clearing heat in all three Burners. In the lower burner it purges the Large Intestine and is commonly used for acute and chronic *constipation* with abdominal pain. In the Middle Burner it smooths the flow of Ki and treats symptoms of stagnation including: fullness, distension and pain of the epigastrium, abdomen, hypochondrium and chest, *nausea* and vomiting, oppression and heaviness of the chest. In the Upper Burner it unblocks the channel pathway and releases exterior heat and wind, treating *pain and inflammation of the throat*, *ear*, *eye*, *arm*, *axilla*, and skin including tinnitus and deafness, headache, redness of the eyes, herpes zoster, intercostal neuralgia, urticaria and other skin diseases.

Treatment
Similar to TH-5.

Triple Heater-10
In the depression of the olecranon fossa of the humerus, about 1" superior to the tip of the olecranon process when the elbow is flexed.

Applications
TH-10 is primarily used for *problems of the elbow*, *especially if there is difficulty in extension* of the forearm.

Treatment
Pressure should be applied perpendicular to the olecranon fossa. A spreading sensation should be felt going deep into the elbow and up the arm.

Triple Heater-14
In the depression posterior and inferior to the acromion, between the posterior and middle belly of the deltoid muscle, approximately 1" posterior to LI-I5. Locate with the arm slightly abducted.

Applications
This is an excellent point for *many shoulder problems* and it is often combined with LI-15 and GB-21.

Treatment
Pressure and stretching techniques are best applied to TH-14 in a sitting or sidelying position.

Triple Heater-16
In the depression on the posterior border of sternocleidomastoid muscle, posterior and approximately 1" inferior to the mastoid process. It is directly below GB-12, on the line joining SI-17, Bl-10 and Du-15.

Applications
TH-16 is an effective point for problems of the ears, neck and entire head. It has the function of clearing wind, heat or dampness and reducing swelling. Common symptoms it is used for include: pain and inflammation of the ears and eyes, deafness, tinnitus, blocked nose, swelling of the face and throat and swollen glands. TH-16 also treats stiffness of the neck with difficulty rotating and side flexing the cervical spine due to tightness of the musculature (commonly on one side only).

Treatment
Shiatsu is best applied with the tips of the fingers in a supine position (without a cushion under the head), or, in a sitting position with the forehead supported by the practitioner so that the muscles of the neck can be relaxed. A sensation should be felt radiating into the head, neck, ears, face and temporal region. **Caution**: Great care should be taken when working on the neck so as to avoid overstimulation or over stretching the area. This is particularly important in elderly or very weak patients and those suffering from hypertension, arthritis or osteoporosis of the spine.

Triple Heater-17
In a deep depression directly behind the ear lobe. Midway between the mandible and the mastoid process, superior to the transverse process of the Atlas (C-1).

Applications
TH-17 may be the most important point for problems of the ear due to it's powerful action on clearing heat and wind of both exterior and interior origin and stopping pain by clearing the channel pathway. It is effectively used in a wide variety of conditions affecting the ear including: *tinnitus*, diminished hearing, *deafness, earache, acute or chronic otitis*, itching, discharge and other inflammatory conditions of the ear. For this purpose it is often combined with other surrounding points including TH-16, GB-2, SI-19 and TH-21. Due to the fact that TH-17 subdues internal wind from the head, it may treat stubborn and difficult conditions such as *Meniere's disease*, dizziness, loss of balance, vertigo, blurred vision, *stiffness of the jaw*, sore throat, headache, sudden deafness, extreme ear pain or tinnitus with dizziness and nausea due to Liver Yang or phlegm-fire rising upwards. TH-17 is also very effective in the treatment of problems of the facial nerve (which emerges deep to TH-17, at the stylomastoid foramen) including *paralysis and/or pain of the face* (jaw, mouth, tongue, cheek and eye), trigemminal neuralgia and difficulty speaking or swallowing.

Treatment
Pressure is best applied with the fingers perpendicular to TH-17 with the ear lobe folded forward. A distending and maybe sore sensation should be felt spreading inwards, around the ear, into the throat and up the sides of the face. Moxa may also be effectively applied for certain conditions including deafness, diminished hearing, stiffness of the jaw, and paralysis of the face and tongue, but only when caused by wind and cold invasions of the channel or extreme deficiency of Ki and Blood. **Caution**: Moxa should **not be used if there is inflammation**. It is normal that a slight sore feeling of the surrounding area may be felt for a couple of hours after strong stimulation has been applied to TH-17.

Triple Heater-20
Directly above the ear apex, within the hairline of the temple. Locate by folding the ear forward. See also GB-8.

Applications and treatment
Similar to TH-18 and TH-19.

Triple Heater-21
In the depression anterior to the supratragic notch and superior to the condyloid process of the mandible appearing when the mouth is opened.

Applications
TH-21 is primarily used for problems of the ear including otitis, tinnitus, deafness and Meniere's disease, but also for other problems of the local area including temporal headache, toothache, facial pain and inflammation of the eyes (see also GB-2 and SI-19).

Treatment
Acupressure is best applied with the mouth slightly open.

Triple Heater-22
Anterior and superior to TH-21, on the course of the superficial temporal artery.

Triple Heater-23
In the depression at the lateral end of the eyebrow.

Applications and treatment
Similar to GB-1.

THE GALLBLADDER CHANNEL
Lesser Yang channel of the lower limb

Gall Bladder-1

In the small depression on the lateral aspect of the orbit, approximately 0.5" lateral to the outer canthus.

Applications

GB-1 *clears the vision and brightens the eyes* and is often combined with distal points such as GB-37 and Liv-3 for this purpose (see also Bl-1 and St-1).

Treatment

Acupressure is applied regularly to GB-1 and other local points including Bl-1, St-1 and Tai Yang.

Gall Bladder-2

In the depression anterior to the intertragic notch, directly below SI-19, at the posterior border of the condyloid process of the mandible. Locate with the mouth slightly open.

Applications

GB-2 is an important point for *problems of the ear* including tinnitus, *itching or pain of the ear,* otitis, parotitis and loss of hearing due to Liver Yang rising, heat or phlegm accumulation.

Treatment

Acupressure is applied regularly until symptoms subside.

Gall Bladder-8

Approximately 1" superior to the apex of the ear, 1.5" within the hairline. Fold the ear forward carefully to locate the apex precisely. Clench the teeth to define the depression of the point.

Applications

GB-8 is a major point to treat the head, particularly because it also has the function of clearing heat, wind and excessive yang from the Liver and Gall Bladder. It is primarily used in the treatment of *temporal headache, migraine, inflammation of the eyes*, and other problems of the head including vertigo, Meniere's disease, dizziness, facial paralysis and psychological disorders. It is an empirical point for *food or alcohol* poisoning with symptoms such as vomiting and abdominal distension accompanied by headache and dizziness.

Treatment

Pressure is best applied unilaterally until a sensation is felt spreading out across the whole of the sides of the head, extending to the eyes, neck and throat. **Caution**: avoid excessive pressure on the cranium.

Gall Bladder-12

In the depression directly posterior and inferior to the mastoid process, 0.4" within the hairline, level with Du-16.

Applications

GB-12, like the other points of the base of the cranium, has the function of clearing wind and other pathogenic factors, particularly phlegm and excessive yang from the head. It therefore has a calming effect on the mind and treats conditions such as *headache, insomnia*, mental agitation and paralysis of the face and body. (see also GB-20, Bl-10, Du-16 and Anmian)

Treatment

Pressure is best applied in a sitting or supine position (without a cushion). See also GB-20.

Gall Bladder-13

0.5" within the anterior hairline, 3" lateral to the anterior midline. Two thirds of the distance from Du-24 to St-8.

Gall Bladder-14

In the depression above the midpoint of the eyebrow, one third of the distance from the top of the eyebrow to the anterior hairline (approximately 1").

Applications

GB-14 is an important point for problems of the *forehead and eyes* including *frontal headache, pain and inflammation of the eyes* and eyelids, *excessive lacrimation* and facial paralysis. GB-14 is also used to calm the mind in cases of *anxiety*, restlessness and insomnia.

Treatment

Acupressure is best applied in a supine position.

Gall Bladder-20

In the centre of the largest depression below the occipital bone, between sternocleidomastoid and trapezius muscles. Midway between Du-16 and GB-12.

Applications

GB-20 is a major point for *problems of the head, sense organs, face and neck*. It has the function of 'descending the impure' (i.e. pathogenic factors such as wind and excessive yang) and 'ascending the pure' (i.e. the clear Ki and Blood). Symptoms it treats include *headache and migraine, dizziness,* facial paralysis, temporomandibular syndrome, *stiffness and pain of the neck*, shoulder pain, *pain and inflammation of the eyes or ears*, failing vision or hearing.

Treatment

Shiatsu is best applied with the tips of the fingers in a supine position (without a cushion under the head) or in a sitting position with the forehead supported by the practitioner so that the muscles of the neck can be relaxed. A strong sensation should be felt radiating upwards across the temples to the face and down the neck toward the shoulder. **Caution:** Great care should be taken when working on the neck to avoid overstimulation or over stretching the area. This is particularly important in elderly or very weak patients and those suffering from hypertension, arthritis or osteoporosis of the spine. Overstimulation may in some cases make the person dizzy or nauseous.

Gall Bladder-21

Above the shoulder, on the highest point of the trapezius muscle, midway between the spinous process of the C-7 vertebra and the lateral tip of the acromion.

Applications

GB-21 has a powerful descending effect clearing pathogenic factors from the head and chest. It is commonly used for *stiffness and tension of the shoulders, headache,* temporomandibular syndrome, *migraine*, pain and inflammation of the eyes and ears, dizziness and delayed labour.

Treatment

GB-21 is effectively treated in a sitting position with the practitioner applying pressure with the palms or forearms, by leaning down on top of the shoulders. It may also be effectively treated in a side position so as to avoid excessive pressure on the lower back. **Caution:** GB-21 descends the Ki very strongly and therefore excessive pressure should not be applied on very tired or deficient people. This is particularly true in the sitting position as inappropriate pressure may cause dizziness and even fainting in extreme cases. Avoid downward pressure to this area completely during pregnancy, heavy menstruation and lower back problems.

Gall Bladder-22
On the mid-axillary line 3" below the axilla, in the fifth intercostal space.

Applications
GB-22 is useful in the treatment of *problems of the axillary area*, including painful swelling and inflammation of the skin or glands of the axilla and breast due to heat and dampness.

Treatment
Pressure is best applied in a sidelying position with the arm abducted. **Caution**: GB-22 can be extremely tender on palpation.

Gall Bladder-23
1" anterior to GB-22, in the fifth intercostal space.

Applications and treatment
Similar to GB-22.

Gall Bladder-24
In the seventh intercostal space, inferior and slightly lateral to Liv-14.

Applications
GB-24 is the *Bo point for the Gall Bladder* and is used for any problem of the gallbladder or liver organs. Symptoms it treats include *hypochondrial pain* and distension, hiccup, *nausea*, vomiting and jaundice. Combine with Liv-14, GB-34 and Liv-3.

Treatment
Similar to Liv-14.

Gall Bladder-25
Directly below the free end of the twelfth rib.

Applications
GB-25 is the Bo point for the Kidneys and is used to tonify the Kidneys and Spleen.

Treatment
Similar to Liv-13. **Caution**: GB-25 is often very tender and great care should be taken not to apply excessive pressure. Do not apply excessive pressure to the floating ribs a they can **fracture very easily**. See also Liv-13.

Gall Bladder-26
On the mid-axillary line, below the free end of the eleventh rib, level with the umbilicus.

Applications
GB-26 is one of the most important points of the *Girdle Vessel* and treats symptoms caused by obstruction of the flow of Ki in this channel and accumulation of dampness in the lower burner and uterus. GB-26 is often combined with GB-41 to treat *leucorrhoea*, dysmenorrhoea, irregular menstruation and *abdominal distension and pain spreading to the lower back, hypochondrium and hips*.

Treatment
GB-26 is best accessed in a sidelying position. **Caution**: GB-26 is often tender and great care should be taken not to apply excessively strong pressure.

Gall Bladder-27 and -28
GB-27 is just medial to the ASIS, level with Ren-4 (3" below the umbilicus) and GB-28 is about one finger's breadth below it (about 0.5").

Applications
Both these points, being on the *Girdle Vessel* are useful to aid in unblocking stagnant Ki from the intestines and reproductive organs. Symptoms they treat include: *abdominal pain at the sides*, *abdominal distension*, *chronic appendicitis*, *leucorrhoea*, *irregular menstruation*, chronic constipation or diarrhoea, prolapse of the uterus and *inguinal hernia*.

Treatment
These points are accessed in a supine position. **Caution**: GB-27 and GB-28 are often very tender and should be approached carefully.

Gall Bladder-29
Midway between the ASIS and the tip of the greater trochanter, located with the hip flexed in a sidelying position.

Applications
GB-29 is a very important local point for pain and any problem of the hip including restricted mobility of the lower limbs and sciatica. It is often combined with other local points such as GB-30 and St-31.

Treatment
Shiatsu is best applied in a side position with the hip in flexion. Stretching out of the surrounding area can also be effectively achieved in this position. A strong relieving aching sensation should be felt spreading into and around the hip joint. Pain and stiffness should be diminished after treatment. **Caution**: GB-29 is often tender on pressure.

Gall Bladder-30
Behind the greater trochanter of the femur, one third of the distance between the greater trochanter and sacral hiatus, located with the hip joint flexed.

Applications
GB-30 is a major point used for *many problems of the hip and lower back* areas. The Bladder channel also passes through GB-30. It is often combined with points such as: GB-34, Bl-40, Bl-60 and Bl-23 to treat lower back pain and sciatica, whereas it is combined with GB-29 for problems of the hip.

Treatment
The best position to treat this point is lying on the side. There are many techniques that can be applied to release GB-30 and it's surrounding area, including moxibustion and cupping. Whatever method of treatment is chosen, there should be a relieving sensation (maybe soreness or aching) spreading to the affected areas. Pain and stiffness should be diminished after treatment.

Gall Bladder-31
On the lateral aspect of the thigh, 7" above the transverse popliteal crease.

Applications
GB-31 is a powerful point used in cases of weakness, pain, atrophy and paralysis of the lower limbs.

Treatment
Acupressure and Shiatsu can be applied to GB-31 and the whole of the iliotibial tract in a supine, side or prone position.

Gall Bladder-33
3" above GB-34 in the depression between the tendon of the biceps femoris muscle and lateral femoral condyle, located with the knee flexed. It is lateral to St-35.

Applications
GB-33 is an important local point for *problems of the lateral aspect of the knee.*

Treatment
Pressure is applied until a sensation radiates up and down the channel.

Gall Bladder-34
In the depression anterior and inferior to the head of fibula. Approximately 1" laterosuperior to St-36.

Applications
GB-34 is one of the most important points of the body used primarily to *spread and smooth the flow of Ki* and clear dampness and heat from the Liver and Gall Bladder channel and organ. It is also the *Gathering point for the Sinews* and therefore treats musculoskeletal problems anywhere in the body, including cramping, spasm, tic, tendinitis, arthritis, stiffness, weakness and atrophy of the muscles. Common symptoms it is used for include: *hypochondrial pain*, pain of the breasts, *abdominal pain*, dysmenorrhoea, PMS, *irritability*, *stiffness of the neck and shoulder*, *pain of the knee* and sciatica. GB-34 is often combined with Liv-3 and Liv-14 to treat Liver Ki stagnation leading to hypochondrial pain and irritability.

Treatment
A strong sensation should radiate up and down the channel.

Gall Bladder-35
7" above the tip of the lateral malleolus, on the posterior border of the fibula, level with GB-36, St-39 and Bl-58.

Gall Bladder-36
In front of GB-35, on the anterior border of the fibula, 7" above the tip of the lateral malleolus. Level with GB-35, St-39 and Bl-58.

Gall Bladder-37
5" above the lateral malleolus, on the anterior border of fibula.

Applications
GB-37 is primarily used for problems of the eyes, including: pain, inflammation and redness of the eyes, excessive lacrimation, night blindness and failing vision.

Treatment
Similar to GB-34.

Gall Bladder-39
3" above the lateral malleolus. This point has two locations depending on the tightness of the local musculature: (a) posterior to the fibula in a depression between the tendons of peroneus longus brevis or between the tendons and the bone, or (b) on the anterior border of the fibula (this location is best suited for people with a lot of tightness and jitsu of the Gallbladder channel).

Applications
GB-39 is the *Gathering point for the marrow* and therefore has a close relationship to the Kidney Essence. GB-39 is a very effective point for *spinal problems, particularly of the neck* and is used to treat pain, stiffness or paralysis of the sinews as well as problems of the bones such as osteoporosis causing *sciatica* and *lower back pain.*

Gall Bladder-40
In the centre of the prominent depression, anterior and inferior to the external malleolus, in the depression on the lateral side of the tendons of the peroneus tertius and extensor digitorum longus muscles.

Applications
GB-40 is the Source point for the Gall Bladder and is used to treat deficiency and Ki stagnation of this organ with symptoms such as hypochondrial pain, acid reflux, stiffness and cramping of the muscles as well as psychological inability to make decisions and act with courage.

Treatment
Acupressure should be applied until a sensation spreading around the point and up the channel is achieved.

Gall Bladder-41
In the depression distal to the junction of the fourth and fifth metatarsal bones, lateral to the tendon of the extensor of the small toe.

Applications
GB-41 is the opening *point of the Girdle Vessel* and treats symptoms such as: abdominal, hip and lower back pain, dysmenorrhoea, leucorrhoea, pain and distension of the hypochondrium, breasts and axilla, tightness of the chest, headache and problems of the eyes and ears. GB-41 can be used during pregnancy as a distal point for hip and back problems.

Treatment
Acupressure should be applied until a spreading sensation is achieved. **Caution**: GB-41 can be very tender.

Gall Bladder-43
Proximal to the margin of the web between the fourth and fifth toes.

Gall Bladder-44
On the lateral side of the fourth toe, about 0.1" proximal to the corner of the nail.

THE LIVER CHANNEL
Absolute Yin Channel of the lower limb

Liver-1
On the lateral side of the big toe, midway between the corner of the nail and the centre of the crease at the interphalangeal joint.

Applications
Liv-1 is primarily used to subdue interior wind and restore consciousness.

Treatment
Similar to the other well points.

Liver-2
On the dorsal aspect of the foot, between the first and second toes, approximately 0.5" proximal to the end of the crease of the web between the toes. Proximal to the metatarsophalangeal joint.

Applications
Liv-2 is primarily used to clear heat and fire from the Liver with symptoms such as migraine headache, red, painful eyes, sore throat, soreness of the genital area, excessive uterine bleeding, insomnia and irritability.

Treatment
Acupressure is applied until an intense numb spreading sensation is achieved.

Liver-3
In the depression distal to the junction of the first and second metatarsal bones.

Applications
Liv-3 is one of the most commonly used points with a wide area of applications. It's functions include both dispersal of pathogenic factors such as excessive Yang, interior wind or heat and tonification of the Liver Yin and Blood. Liv-3 has an effect on the whole body by influencing the smooth flow of Ki and Blood, particularly in the head, eyes, chest, stomach, intestines and reproductive system. Common symptoms it is used for include: *headache, migraine, dizziness, vertigo,* epilepsy, TIA,[15] *pain, inflammation and tiredness of the eyes, blurred vision,* failing vision, insomnia, mental restlessness, *irritability, constriction, pain and heaviness of the chest, hypochondrial or epigastric pain,* acid reflux, nausea, *vomiting,* jaundice, *irritable bowel syndrome, abdominal distension and pain, dysmenorrhoea, delayed menstruation and labour, irregular menstruation,* infertility, *genital itching and pain* and *PMS.* Combine Liv-3 with GB-34 for Ki and Blood stagnation in the Liver, with LI-4 to treat stress, tension, pains anywhere in the body and addiction related problems and with Sp-4 and Ren-4 for Blood stasis in the uterus.

Treatment
A strong sensation should be achieved for best results. **Caution**: Liv-3 is a very strong point and can have powerful effects on the mind and body. Care should be taken not to over-stimulate it, particularly in very deficient people, during pregnancy and when there is severe Ki and Blood stagnation.

Liver-4
Anterior to the medial malleolus, level with it's tip when the foot at right angles to the tibia (dorsiflexion) in the depression on the medial side of the tibialis anterior tendon. Midway between Sp-5 and St-41.

Applications
Liv-4 is used for problems of the lower burner including dysmenorrhoea and endometriosis as well as effectively treating *pain, swelling and stiffness of the ankle* and medial aspect of the foot.

Treatment
Similar to Liv-3. **Caution**: Avoid over-stimulation of Liv-5 during pregnancy.

Liver-5
On the medial aspect of the tibia, 5" above the medial malleolus in a small depression just posterior to the medial tibial border.

Applications
Liv-5 has the function of smoothing the flow of Liver Ki and clearing dampness and heat from the lower burner. It is a very important point for problems of the genitourinary organs with symptoms such as: *pain, itching or swelling of the vagina, cervix, urethra, testicles or prostate gland*, lower abdominal pain, *dysuria, leucorrhoea, dysmenorrhoea, insufficient dilation of the cervix during labour*, prolapse of the uterus, *inguinal hernia*, orchitis, torsion of the testicles, *excessive libido* and priapism. It also effectively treats other symptoms of Liver Ki stagnation such as hypochondrial pain, tightness of the chest, plum stone throat, poor vision, depression, mood swings and irritability.

Treatment
Pressure or moxa should be applied directly behind the medial tibial border until a sensation radiates up the medial aspect of the leg and thigh. See also Sp-6.

Liver-6
A little more than half way down the medial aspect of the tibia (approximately 0.5"), posterior to the medial tibial border. 2" above Liv-5 and 7" above the medial malleolus.

Applications
Liv-6 is the *accumulation point of the Liver channel* and therefore treats acute pain of the channel pathway as well as Blood stasis and heat.

Treatment
Similar to Liv-5.

Liver-8
Posterior and superior to the medial end of the popliteal crease, in the depression appearing when the knee is flexed, above the tendons of the semitendinosus and semimembranosus muscles (they insert into the medial aspect of the tibia). If the thumb is placed on Liv-8 the index finger naturally locates Kd-10 which is directly behind the muscles. This illustrates the close relationship between these two channels.

Applications
Liv-8 is a major point to tonify the Liver Blood and Yin, and remove dampness, heat and Blood stasis from the lower burner, particularly the uterus. Common problems it is used for include pain, swelling and itching of the genitals, *dysmenorrhoea*, endometriosis, ovarian cysts, *abdominal distension and pain, leucorrhoea, dysuria*, diarrhoea, headache and *painful swelling of the knee*.

Treatment
Pressure should be applied in the supine position with the knee flexed and well supported with cushions. A distending warmth or sore sensation should extend around the point and/or up and down the channel.

Liver-9
4" above Liv-8, between the vastus medialis and sartorius muscles. When the foot is dorsiflexed a groove appears in this area.

Liver-10
3" below St-30, on the anterior border of the adductor longus muscle.

Liver-11
2" below St-30, on the anterior border of the adductor longus muscle.

Liver-12
At the inguinal groove, just medial to the femoral artery. Lateral and inferior to St-30, 2.5" lateral to the anterior midline at the level of the pubic symphysis. Note that Sp-12 is located about 0.5" lateral to Liv-12, on the lateral side of the femoral artery.

Liver-13
On the lateral side of the abdomen, below the free end of the 11th rib.

Applications
Liv-13 is the *Bo point for the Spleen* and the *Gathering point for the Yin Organs* and has the function of strengthening the middle and lower burners by tonifying and harmonising the Ki. It tonifies the Spleen and regulates the Liver Ki, particularly in relation to the digestive system. It is used to treat many problems of the stomach, spleen, gallbladder, pancreas and intestines with symptoms such as: *indigestion, distension and heaviness of the epigastrium and abdomen, belching*, nausea, *flatulence, loose or bitty stools, diarrhoea* and *constipation*. This is especially evident when the Liver Ki invades the Spleen. Liv-13 also treats other symptoms of Spleen deficiency and stagnation of Ki including *distension and fullness of the chest and hypochondrium*, constriction and heaviness of the chest, dyspnoea and coughing due to Ki stagnation or phlegm-damp accumulation, weakness of the limbs and body, *pain of the lumbar or thoracic spine* with difficulty rotating or side-flexing the trunk and difficulty raising the arm due to contraction of the muscles of the abdomen.

Treatment
Shiatsu is best applied in a supine position with the hips flexed and the legs well supported with cushions, so that the abdomen can be as relaxed as possible. Self-acupressure can also be applied in a standing or sitting position while bending the trunk forward. A warm spreading sensation should be felt radiating upwards under the ribs to the chest and/or across the epigastrium, intestines and entire abdomen. **Caution**: Liv-13 can be very tender and should always be approached carefully; palm pressure is applied initially, before other 'tools of shiatsu' such as the thumbs or fingers are used. Avoid pressure on Liv-13 (and other abdominal points) if the abdomen is very painful and hard in cases of severe constipation or inflammation of the abdomen. Do not apply excessive pressure to the floating ribs a they can **fracture very easily**.

Liver-14
Directly below the root of the breast, on the midmammilary line, in the sixth intercostal space.

Applications
Liv-14 is a very important point as it is the *Bo point for the Liver*. It is used when there is stagnation of Ki and Blood in the chest, liver or digestive system. It is also used to cool the Blood.

Treatment
Acupressure should be applied until a distending sensation is felt spreading out across the chest and epigastrium and into the thoracic cavity toward the liver, spleen, stomach, diaphragm and lungs.

THE DIRECTING (CONCEPTION) VESSEL
Ocean of Yin

Ren-1
In the centre of the perineum, midway between the genitals and the anus.

Applications and treatment
Ren-1 has the functions of nourishing the Yin and benefiting the Essence, resolving dampness and heat from the lower burner and promoting resuscitation. The *Penetrating, Governing and Conception Vessels* meet at Ren-1, which is considered as opposite to Du-20 both in function and location (Du-20 tonifies and raises the Yang Ki). Ren-1 is used in many Qigong exercises as a point to contain and gather the Yin energies of the body. It is unfortunate that due to its location, Ren-1 is not very commonly used.

Ren-2
On the anterior midline, 5" below the umbilicus, just above the pubic symphysis.

Applications and treatment
Similar to Ren-3, but not as strong.

Ren-3
On the anterior midline, 4" below the umbilicus.

Applications
Ren-3 is the *Bo point for the Bladder* and is primarily used for problems of the genitourinary system. Common symptoms it is used for include: *dysuria, frequent urination, lower abdominal pain and distension, leucorrhoea, genital itching and pain*, uterine prolapse, infertility, *dysmenorrhoea* and irregular menstruation.

Treatment
Pressure is best applied in a supine position with the hips flexed and the legs well supported with cushions, so that the abdomen can be as relaxed as possible. A spreading sensation should be achieved around the point and down towards the perineum. Moxa is very effective to clear dampness and cold from the lower burner and tonify the Yang Ki. **Caution**: Avoid pressure on Ren-3 (and other abdominal points) if the abdomen is very painful and hard in cases of severe constipation, inflammation of the abdomen or pregnancy.

Ren-4
On the anterior midline, 3" below the umbilicus.

Applications
Ren-4 is the *Bo point for the Small Intestine and intersection of the Liver, Spleen and Kidneys*. It therefore has the function of strengthening these organs, particularly in relation to the reproductive organs, urinary system and intestines. Ren-4 is called the *Gate of the Original Ki* (similar to Bl-26, the yu point for the *Original Ki Gate*) as it has a direct effect on the Kidneys and entire lower burner. It particularly tonifies the Yin, Blood and Essence and calms and roots the shen (it is often combined with Sp-6 for this purpose). Common complaints it is used for include: *irregular menstruation, amenorrhoea, infertility, fibroids or cysts of the ovaries and uterus*, endometriosis, *dysmenorrhoea*, dysuria, *leucorrhoea, abdominal distension*, irritable bowel, anxiety, *restlessness, insomnia, heat due to Yin deficiency*, sore throat and *emaciation of the flesh*.

Treatment
Similar to Ren-3. Moxa can also be applied to tonify the Yang Ki and dispel cold from the lower burner.

Ren-5
On the anterior midline, 2" below the umbilicus.

Applications
Ren-5 is the *Bo for the Triple Heater* and is used for weakness of the fluid transformation in the lower burner.

Treatment
Similar to Ren-3.

Ren-6
On the anterior midline, 1.5" below the umbilicus.

Applications
Ren-6 is the point of *the Sea of Ki* (similarly to Bl-24) and is used to treat deficiency of Ki and Yang and stagnation of Ki in the abdomen. It is commonly combined with St-36 for *general weakness*, with Sp-3 and Ren-12 for weakness of the Stomach and Spleen and with St-36 and Du-20 for *sinking Ki*.

Treatment
Similar to Ren-3.

Ren-8
On the anterior midline, in the centre of the umbilicus.

Applications
Ren-8 restores collapsed Yang with symptoms such as *diarrhoea*, *general weakness* with profuse sweating.

Treatment
Similar to Ren-3. Moxa should be applied. **Caution**: although pressure can be applied to the umbilicus, it is often tender and special care should be taken to ensure the correct angle and depth. A sensation of warmth should be felt in the whole abdomen after treatment.

Ren-9
On the anterior midline, 1" above the umbilicus.

Applications
Ren-9 is primarily used to aid in fluid transformation and treats *oedema* and *swelling*.

Treatment
See Ren-3 and Ren-12. A spreading sensation should be achieved around the point and down the channel.

Ren-10
On the anterior midline, 2" above the umbilicus.

Applications
Ren-10 has the primary function of aiding the descending of Stomach Ki when there are symptoms of indigestion nausea, acid reflux, fullness of the epigastrium and abdomen, foul breath and belching. It has a particular effect on the *lower part of the stomach* therefore relieving food retention. Ren-10 also tonifies the Spleen Ki.

Treatment
Similar to Ren-9 and Ren-12.

Ren-12
On the anterior midline, 4e above the umbilicus.

Applications
Ren-12, being the *Bo point for the Stomach* is a very important point to tonify the middle burner's Ki and is used in many conditions caused by deficiency of the Spleen and Stomach. Symptoms include: *poor appetite and digestion, nausea, productive cough, morning sickness during pregnancy, fullness and heaviness of the epigastrium, loose stools, poor concentration, restlessness and tiredness*. Ren-12 is primarily used for deficiency conditions and particularly affects the *middle part of the stomach*, in which case it is often combined with St-36, Sp-6, Sp-3 and Bl-20 and Bl-21. Ren-12 also nourishes the Yin and body fluids because the *Stomach is the origin of fluids and Yin* (whereas the Kidneys are the Root of Yin). In cases of *thirst, dry mouth*, sore throat, scant urination and *other symptoms of dryness* combine Ren-12 with St-36 and Kd-6.

Treatment
Similar to Ren-9. Moxa is also applied to dispel cold from the stomach and tonify the Spleen yang. **Caution**: Avoid excessive pressure on the epigastrium. Always apply pressure here very carefully;the palms should be used initially.

Ren-13
On the anterior midline, 5" above the umbilicus.

Applications and treatment
Similar to Ren-12, but more for acute cases, particularly nausea and vomiting. Ren-13 particularly affects the *upper part of the stomach.*

Ren-14
On the anterior midline, 6" above the umbilicus, below the tip of the xiphoid process. Location varies depending on the length of the xiphoid process.

Applications
Ren-14 is the *Bo point for the Heart* and is used to treat symptoms of heat and stagnation of the Heart and chest including *palpitations, dyspnoea*, coughing, pain and *constriction of the chest and epigastrium*, insomnia, anxiety and *emotional upsets in general*. Ren-14 also descends rebellious Stomach Ki in cases of *nausea and vomiting.*

Treatment
Similar to Ren-12. A spreading sensation (maybe sore or electric) is felt going down the channel toward the abdomen and into the thoracic cavity toward the diaphragm and heart. **Caution**: Never press too hard directly onto the xiphoid process, as it can **fracture very easily**.

Ren-15
7" above the umbilicus at the tip of, or on the xyphoid process. Location varies depending on the length of the xiphoid process.

Applications and treatment
Similar to Ren-14. Ren-15 is the *Connecting point for the Directing Vessel* and has the function of freeing up the whole abdomen when there is blockage of the Ki. It also tonifies all the Yin organs and original Ki.

Ren-17
At the centre of the chest, on the anterior midline, level with the fourth intercostal space, between the nipples.

Applications
Ren-17 is a major point to tonify and regulate the chest and is used for problems of this area. Ren-17 is the *Bo point for the Heart Protector*, *the Gathering point for Ki and point of the Upper Sea of Ki (Ren-6 is the point of the Lower sea of Ki)* Common symptoms it is used for include constriction, tightness, pain or heaviness of the chest, frequent sighing, plum stone throat, cough, dyspnoea, asthma, insufficient lactation and pain of the breasts. It may also be thought of as the *Bo point for the Shen* as it is used to treat many emotional disorders including depression, propensity for crying, hysteria, insomnia and bereavement. Ren-17 is often combined with HP-6.

Treatment
Very gentle pressure should be used initially. **Caution**: Do not apply excessive pressure to the chest.

Ren-22
On the anterior midline in the centre of the suprasternal notch.

Applications
Ren-22 is primarily used to descend rebellious Ki with symptoms such as coughing, wheezing and dyspnoea.

Treatment
Pressure is applied downwards so that a spreading sensation goes down into the chest. **Caution**: Do not press perpendicularly to the throat, for obvious reasons.

Ren-23
On the anterior midline, above the Adam's Apple, in the depression at the upper border of the hyoid bone.

Applications
Ren-23 is employed in problems of the tongue, throat and submandibular glands.

Treatment
Similar to Ren-23.

Ren-24
In the depression at the centre of the mentolabial groove.

Applications
Ren-24 is effective in treatment of *paralysis of the mouth*, facial pain and problems of the gums, teeth and salivary glands.

Treatment
Acupressure is applied gently until a spreading out sensation is achieved.

GOVERNING VESSEL
Ocean of Yang

Du-1

Midway between the tip of the coccyx and the anus.

Applications

Du-1 is primarily used for problems of the anus and rectum including haemorrhoids and prolapse. It also regulates and tonifies the Ki of the spine and the Yang of the whole body because it is the *Connecting point of the Governing Vessel*. It also calms the mind.

Treatment

Pressure is best applied with the palms or feet. **Caution**: avoid placing the hands and fingers on the area in an 'indiscreet' way. **Do not apply excessive pressure on the coccyx**.

Du-2

On the posterior midline at the sacral hiatus.

Du-4

On the posterior midline below the spinous process of L2.

Applications

Du-4 is one of the most powerful points to tonify the Kidney Essence and Kidney Yang, being located at 'the Gate of Vitality'. Moxibustion is very useful in these cases. Du-4 is often combined with Bl-23, Bl-52 and Kd-3 to tonify the Kidneys.

Treatment

Pressure is best applied perpendicularly to the space between the spinous processes with the thumbs or finger tips. Alternatively, pressure can be applied bilaterally inward toward the spine in cases where the point is too tight due to malformation or injury to the vertebrae. **Contra-indicated** for moxibustion on patients younger than 20 years of age. This is because it powerfully tonifies the Yang Ki, which in younger people, could have the effect of over heating the body.

Du-10

On the posterior midline below the spinous process of T6.

Applications

Similar to Bl-16, the Yu point for the Governing Vessel. See also page 231.

Treatment

See Du-4.

Du-14

On the posterior midline below the spinous process of C7.

Applications

Du-14 is the intersection of the all the Yang channels and therefore has the function of tonifying or sedating the Yang Ki and regulating the ascending and descending of Yang Ki. It clears heat and subdues wind. It also releases the exterior in cases of wind-heat and wind-cold.

Treatment

Pressure is best applied in a sitting position. Cups and moxa can also be used.

Du-15
On the posterior midline, 0.5" below Du-16 in the depression 0.5" within the hairline.

Du-16
Directly below the external occipital protuberance, in the depression between the attachments of the trapezius muscle.

Du-20
On the mid-saggital line, on the midpoint of the line connecting the apex of the two ears. 7" above the posterior hairline, 5" behind the anterior hairline. Fold the ear forward carefully to locate the apex precisely.

Applications
Du-20 is considered the most Yang point of the body (in this respect it is opposite to Ren-1 and Kd-1) and has the function of subduing excessive Yang and interior wind from the head with symptoms such as: headache, dizziness, agitation, epilepsy, loss of consciousness, tinnitus and visual impairment. Du-20 also has the crucial action of raising the Yang Ki when it is very deficient and sinks downwards causing problems such as prolapse of the uterus or rectum, haemorrhoids, chronic diarrhoea, poor concentration and mental exhaustion.

Treatment
Pressure can be applied in a sitting or supine position.

Du-23
1" within the anterior hairline.

Applications
Du-23 is particularly beneficial for problems of nose and sinuses.

Treatment
Acupressure is applied until the nose has opened.

Du-24
0.5" within the anterior hairline.

Du-25
At the tip of the nose.

Du-26
Below the nose, about one third of the distance between the bottom of the nose and the top of the lip, a little above the midpoint of the philtrum.

Applications
This is the most important point to revive consciousness and restore Yin-Yang harmony.

Treatment
Apply strong prerssure with your thumbnail until consciousness is restored.

Du-28
Between the upper lip and upper labial gingiva, in the frenulum of the upper lip.

Classification
Intersection of the Governing Vessel with the Directing Vessel and Stomach channel.

NON CHANNEL POINTS
Extra Points

HEAD AND NECK
Yin Tang *'Imprint Hall'*
Midway between the medial ends of the eyebrows.

Applications
Yin Tang is an important point to *calm the mind* and *stop pain of the frontal area* of the face. It has a beneficial effect on the *sinuses, eyes and nose*. It also regulates the endocrine system by stimulating the hypophysis and pineal gland which are located directly behind the point.

Treatment
Acupressure is applied gently until a sensation (often like 'cool water) is felt going into the head.

Tai Yang *'The Sun'*
In the depression about I" posterior to the midpoint between the outer canthus of the eye and the tip of the eyebrow.

Applications
Tai Yang is an extremely useful point for temporal headache, migraine and pain of the eyes.

Treatment
Acupressure is applied regularly until a cute symptoms subside. Pain should be reduced after treatment.

Yu Yao *'Fish's Lumbus'*
In the middle of the eyebrow, directly above the pupil.

Applications
Yu Yao is an excellent point for many problems of the eyes.

Treatment
Acupressure is applied regularly until the eyes have cleared. Discomfort should be reduced after treatment.

Bi Tong *'Nose Passage'*
In the depression below the nasal bone, at the superior end of the nasolabial sulcus.

Applications
Similar to LI-20, but more effective when the sinuses are also blocked.

Treatment
Acupressure is applied regularly until the nose has unblocked and the breathing is easier.

Anmian *'Peaceful Sleep'*
On the posterior border of mastoid process, midway between GB-20 and TH-17.

Applications
Anmian is primarily used for the treatment of insomnia and has similar functions to GB-12.

Treatment
Acupressure is applied until the whole body relaxes.

Bai Lao *'Hundred Labours'*
One third of the way down the neck, 1" lateral to the posterior midline. 1" inferior to the posterior hairline and 2" superior to the lower border of the spinous process of the C7 vertebra.

Applications
Bai Lao is used when there is depletion of the vital substances and exhaustion with difficulty keeping the head upright, poor concentration and pain, paralysis or stiffness of the neck. It also effectively treats symptoms of phlegm accumulation and deficiency of Ki in the Lungs with symptoms such as dyspnoea, spontaneous sweating, night sweating, cough and lymphadenopathy. It can be combined with Sp-21, LI-4 and Liv-3 for pains throughout the whole body.

Treatment
A strong sensation should be felt going up and down the channel, around the neck and down towards the chest.

BACK, WAIST AND ABDOMEN
Ding Chuan *'Calm Asthma'*
0.5" lateral to Du-14.

Applications
Ding Chuan is primarily used in the treatment of wheezing, dyspnoea cough and asthma.

Treatment
Similar to the upper Yu points.

Hua Tuo Jiaji *'Hua Tuo's Paravertebral Points'*
In the groove closest to the cervical, thoracic and lumbar spine, where they are felt to be most reactive. 0.5" to 1" lateral to either the lower borders or the tips of the spinous processes of the vertebrae.

Applications and treatment
Similar to the Yu points. They are very effective for spinal problems.

Shi Qi Zhui *'Seventeenth Vertebra point'*
On the posterior midline, between the fifth lumbar vertebra and the sacrum.

Applications
Shi Qi Zhui is very effective to treat pain and weakness of the lumbo-sacral joint. It is also effective for acute dysmenorrhoea.

Treatment
Pressure is best applied in a prone position with cushions under the abdomen so that the pelvis is raised and the lumbo-sacral joint opens up.

Zi Gong *'Child's Palace'*
3" lateral to Ren-3, 4" below the umbilicus.

Applications
Zi Gong is primarily used for problems of the ovaries and uterus, including infertility, leucorrhoea, irregular menstruation, functional uterine bleeding and abdominal pain.

UPPER LIMB
Jian Nei Ling *'Front of the Shoulder'*
Midway between the anterior axillary fold and LI- 15, located with the arm adducted.

Applications

This is a very useful point for stiffness and pain of the shoulder, particularly when there is difficulty adducting the arm.

Luo Zhen *'Crick in the Neck'*

Between the second and third metacarpal bones about 0. 5" proximal to the metacarpophalangeal joints, where it is felt most tender.

Applications

Luo Zhen is primarily used to release neck pain and stiffness.

Treatment

A strong aching sensation should be felt spreading up the dorsum of the hand and up the arm to the shoulder and neck.

Yao Tong Dian *'Lumbar Pain Point'*

Two points on the dorsum of the hand, 1" distal to the wrist crease, one point between the second and third and one point between the fourth and fifth metacarpals.

Applications

Yao Tong is used mainly for acute backache and sprain of the lumbus.

Treatment

Similar to Luo Zhen.

Ba Xie *'Eight evils'*

Eight points, on the webs between the fingers of each hand, fist clenched.

Applications

These points are used to treat problems of the fingers such as arthritis, swelling and contracture of the fingers. They also affect the head and face and are used to treat headache, earache, pain of the eyes and fever.

Treatment

Acupressure is applied until a numbness spreads to the surrounding area. Pain and stiffness should be reduced after treatment.

Si Feng *'Four seams'*

Four points in the midpoint of the transverse creases of the proximal interphalangeal joints of the second to fifth digits, on the palmar aspect of the hands.

Applications

These points are primarily used in children and babies and to treat malnutrition. Their function is to tonify the digestive system and improve the Spleenfs transformation and transportation of food essences and body fluids. Symptoms include emaciation, swelling of the abdomen, diarrhoea, vomiting, lack of appetite, colic and respiratory problems such as cough and asthma.

LOWER LIMB
Xiyan *'Eyes of the Knee'*

A pair of points, one in the medial and one in the lateral depression formed by the patellar ligament when the knee is flexed (St-35 forms the lateral point of the pair).

Applications
These points are excellent for any problems of the knee, particularly pain.

Treatment
Pressure is applied perpendicularly to the joint space, between the femur and tibia so that a spreading sensation is felt. Pain and stiffness should be reduced after treatment.

Dan Nang Xue *'Gallbladder Point'*
About 1" below GB-34 in the most painful spot.

Applications
This point is used for problems of the gallbladder including gallstones and inflammation. Symptoms include: nausea, poor digestion of fats, obesity and acute pain of the hypochondrial area.

Lan Wei Xue *'Appendix Point'*
About 2" below St-36 in the most painful spot.

Applications
This point is used to treat chronic appendicitis.

Ba Feng *'Eight winds'*
Eight points altogether located on the dorsal aspect of the feet between the toes, proximal to the margin of the webs.

Applications
These points have the function of clearing heat, descending rebellious Yang and stopping pain.

NOTES

1. 'Tsubo', 'point', 'acu-point' are all terms referring to the same thing.
2. also known as *moxa*
3. The Savior General Compendium, p.29, Ellis, Wiseman, Boss, *Fundamentals of Chinese Acupuncture*, Paradigm Publications, Massachusetts, 1991
4. Classic of difficulties, chapter 27, quoted from p.355, Giovanni Maciocia, *The Foundations of Chinese Medicine*, Churchill Livingston, 1989
5. This highlights the importance the kidneys play in the body's protection (being Extraordinary Vessels they are directly related to the kidneys)
6. i.e. the Gathering Ki
7. All the *well* points (except for HP-9 and Liv-1) are located at the junction of the line drawn along the medial or lateral border of the nail and along the base of the nail.
8. As first aid only.
9. As first aid only.
10. These points (see also BI-26, BI-29, BI-30) are not actually classified as *Yu points* but their name suggests that they are related to the substance or area mentioned.
11. as above for BI-24
12. as above for BI-24.
13. as above for BI-24.
14. The Terminal Yin channels are the Heart Protector and Liver
15. Transient ischaemic attach.

Useful Addresses

The European Shiatsu School can be contacted at:

The European Shiatsu School,
Central Administration,
High Banks,
Lockeridge,
Marlborough,
Wilts., SN8 4EQ
England

Tel: +44(0)1672 513444
e-mail: info@shiatsu.org.uk

www.shiatsu.org.uk

Index